THE GENERAL PRACTICE MANAGEMENT HANDBOOK

The Management of Health Care

Series Editors
John J. Glynn and David A. Perkins

Published:

Managing Health Care

Edited by John J. Glynn and David A. Perkins

The Clinician's Management Handbook

Eidted by David M. Hansell and Brian Salter

Achieving Value for Money

Edited by John J. Glynn, David A. Perkins and Simon Stewart

THE GENERAL PRACTICE MANAGEMENT HANDBOOK

Edited by

Peter Orton

General Practitioner, Hatfield Heath, Essex
Senior Lecturer, University of Bath

and

Claire Hill

Senior Lecturer
Anglia Business School, Anglia University

WB Saunders Company Ltd
London   Philadelphia   Toronto   Sydney   Tokyo

W. B. Saunders Company Ltd 24–28 Oval Road
London NW1 7DX

The Curtis Center
Independence Square West
Philadelphia, PA 19106–3399, USA

Harcourt Brace & Company
55 Horner Avenue
Toronto, Ontario M8Z 4X6, Canada

Harcourt Brace & Company, Australia
30–52 Smidmore Street
Marrickville, NSW 2204, Australia

Harcourt Brace & Company, Japan
Ichibancho Central Building, 22–1 Ichibancho
Chiyoda-ku, Tokyo 102, Japan

This publication aims to provide accurate, authoritative information
and comment on the subjects it covers. It is sold on the understanding
that the publisher is not in business as a lawyer or consultant.

This book is printed on acid free paper

A catalogue record of this book is available from the British Library

ISBN 0-7020-2204-7

Typeset by Paston Press Ltd, Loddon, Norfolk
Printed and bound in Great Britain by WBC, Bridgend, Mid Glamorgan

CONTENTS

CONTRIBUTORS

Karen Bloor   Research Fellow, Department of Health Services Clinical Evaluation, The University of York, UK

Paul Chapman   BA, MBA, Managing Director of Organisation Improvement Change Management Consultancy

Roger Higgs   Professor of General Practice, Kings College Medical School, London, UK

Peter Hildebrand   MA (Cantab), Solicitor, Chairman of Industrial Tribunals, Leeds Region, UK

Claire Hill   MA, DipIMD, MIPD, Senior Lecturer, Anglia Business School, Chelmsford, UK

Ivan Lester   BPharm, MRPharmS, Director, Harrogate Public Sector Management Centre Ltd, Ripley Castle, Harrogate, UK

Alan Maynard   Professor of Economics, University of York, UK

Peter Orton   FRCGP, MMed Sci, General Practitioner, Hatfield Heath, Essex, UK, Senior Lecturer, Centre for Continuing Education, Bath University, UK

Tony Rennison   BSc, PhD, CChem, MRSC, Independent Medical Computing Consultant, GP Tutor, TPMDE, Millman St, London, UK

Carolyn Semple Piggot   MRPharmS, MIIS, Editorial board member for *Journal of Managed Care*, Syndicate leader for the PMCPA study days, Business development manager, Glaxo Wellcome Healthcare Ltd, Uxbridge, UK

Laurence Slavin   ACA, Chartered Accountant, Adviser to NHS Executive on GPs finances, Ramsay Brown and Partners, London, UK

FOREWORD

Denis Pereira Gray

There are many reasons why management in primary care is becoming steadily more important. First, the size of practices continues to increase through the average number of partners; secondly and separately the size of the team has grown with counsellors, district nurses, midwives, physiotherapists, practice managers, practice nurses all now commonly members of the extended primary care team.

These structural changes have all arisen as a response to the growing complexity of the work. These arise from the introduction of new drugs, new treatments, and new ways of working – all highlighted by a continuing fall in the average duration of stay by patients in hospital and the rise in the numbers of patients receiving day care surgery

These changes create new management issues which all need solving at once. Hence the call both for more management input and greater skills. Professional bodies such as the Royal College of General Practitioners (RCGP) and the Association of Practice Managers (AMGP) are emphasising the importance of management and new forms of accreditation and quality assurance in primary care.

The General Practice Management Handbook has an interesting approach in that it concentrates on broad principles rather than detail. The bulk of the book is concerned with the management of people both as individuals and as teams, and as the main resource within a practice to achieve plans and objectives. It is written to appeal to all concerned with management including those doctors, like some of the authors, who have an interest. It is particularly strong on scene setting – not just in the UK, but also in an international context – and tackles difficult but important issues such as negotiation skills and obtaining value for money, which transcend day-to-day activities. There are also useful chapters on statutory responsibilities, ethics and IT.

A multidisciplinary approach is the new theme in primary care and the multidisciplinary authorship of this book reflect this by including contributions from: an accountant, a business school academic, a computing consultant, doctors, health economists, a lawyer, and a pharmacist.

At a time of rapid change in primary care, with three White Papers and the 1997 Primary Care Act in the last 12 months alone, and many more changes soon to come, this is a helpful addition to the literature in a fast expanding field.

Professor Denis Pereira Gray OBE MA FRCGP Hon FRSH
Director of the Postgraduate Medical School
Professor of General Practice, University of Exeter
General Practitioner, Exeter

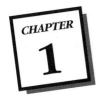

RESPONDING TO THE CHANGING NATURE OF PRIMARY CARE

Peter Orton

Peter Orton

OBJECTIVES

> ◆ To understand the changes taking place in the UK health care system.
>
> ◆ To identify the impact these changes will have on primary care and in particular on the primary health care team.
>
> ◆ To explore the new role and skills required to meet these changes and the value of effective management within primary care.

INTRODUCTION

Western health care systems are going through a time of rapid change and these changes will affect all those involved in providing health care. Systems are facing pressure to spend more as demand for health care services increases. As a result, the principle of managed care is being established to contain costs, and a dilemma is created between the managers wanting value for money and the doctors who want to provide care with little consideration of the cost. This managed service is already evident in both secondary and primary care. As managed care develops, so health care professionals will become increasingly accountable for their use of limited resources. This value-for-money approach will become linked to the quality of care provided. Currently the quality of care is inconsistent and it is this variation that will have to be reduced.

Primary care will need to be able to adapt to the process of continual change and to make effective use of resources. This has become part of modern health care. For those able to anticipate and handle change, there are many opportunities but for those unprepared the process will be difficult.

Additional skills will be required in order to face these challenges effectively in the areas of management, quality assurance, needs assessment and ethics. As primary care moves further towards a regulated health market, it will be those practices with effective management that will be successful in providing care within the available resources.

PRESENT STATE OF UK HEALTH CARE

In the UK, health care expenditure is significantly lower than the level of national income would suggest, on the basis of other countries' expenditures. It is likely that this level of public expenditure on health will remain unaltered. The UK's spending on health has decreased over the last 30 years when compared to many other Western countries. The percentage of gross domestic product (GDP) spent on health in 1994 was 6.9%. This was well below the average for the OECD (Organisation of Economic Co-operation and Development) countries and the lowest of the G7 group of leading industrialized nations. The pressure on resources appears to be greater in the UK than that experienced by other OECD countries. UK health care funding may be inadequate. Relative underfunding of the system means that the provision of care will be limited and difficult choices, as to the level of need to be met, will have to be made.

The problem is further compounded by the fact that it is difficult to provide a complete package of care for the individual. The funding of health and social care has remained separate, and is unlikely to change in the foreseeable future. The funding of social services by local government and health care by the NHS has resulted in separate services. The separation of social and medical services has meant that caring for patients' different needs, in primary care, has been difficult.

Present principles of health care

Traditionally these principles have been those of availability and accessibility. It is only recently that accountability has been added. Availability is the provision of a service, and health care services have largely been available. Most services have been provided at little cost to the user. It is only recently that some services are no longer available or have a low priority in their provision. Examples include specialist infertility services, cosmetic surgery and sterilization. Accessibility is the ease of use of a service. Accessible services have been provided with few barriers to accessing them. While this principle is still true for health care, it is now different for social care. Access to social care is based on a needs-led assessment with some services only accessible to those most in need. Accountability to the consumer and management has developed and includes three elements (Health Policy and Economic Research Unit, 1994a). These are giving accounts of actions, being held to account for them and taking account of the views of those on whose behalf management of a service is being carried out.

Trends in health care   There are a number of trends in health care that are influencing primary care. These influences mean the system has to change. However, the changes are more complex and are moving more rapidly than previously. As a result, the health service of the future will have to be more cost effective, responsive to change and accountable for its use of resources and quality of services. The Welsh Health Planning Forum (1994) identified two possible outcomes from these trends, one desirable and the other undesirable. Each outcome would have a different impact on primary care. The influences on health care are shown in Box 1.1.

Box 1.1
Influences on health care

♦ Demography and epidemiology

♦ Lifestyle factors

♦ Social trends

♦ Economy and working conditions

♦ Science and technology

♦ Health and social policy

♦ Prevalence of disease.

1. Demography and epidemiology
The number of people in the population continues to increase slowly; many are living longer and whilst still suffering from long-term illness. In particular the number of elderly will expand rapidly. More people will reach old age as many of the causes of premature death, death before the age of 65, now have a reduced effect. An additional factor is the reduction of the fertility rate. The overall effect is an increased dependency on the working population as shown by changes in the dependency ratio, the proportion of those not working to those working. The UK ratio is now well above the average for other European countries.

This older population will have an increased demand for health care, the costs of providing this health care will continue to rise and the pressure on the working population will increase. Solutions will include improvements in the efficiency of the health system, greater community support and flexibility in the services themselves. Health care must aim to provide effective health promotion and reduce morbidity.

2. Lifestyle factors
Healthy lifestyles are important in the prevention of many common illnesses. The large beneficial changes in lifestyle expected by many health planners either may not occur or may do so at a reduced

rate. The result will be a continuing demand on health care. Even if there was a reduction through health promotion, this may not have an effect, as more people will be alive and live longer. Health promotion will be required with delivery through primary care. Health care must aim to reduce harmful behaviours.

3. Social trends

Family stability is fragmenting. The divorce rate is high, births outside marriage are increasing, more women are working and the proportion of people living alone is increasing rapidly. Unemployment is likely to increase and families will live further apart. The preferred form of transport is shifting towards a private system. This will be most disadvantageous to older people and the poorest quintile of households. The effect will be the loss of communities and the support that they provide, particularly for the informal carers. Family instability and the increasing isolation of many will add further to people's stress and cause further ill-health. Education on health matters will increase people's expectations, and create further demands on services and their quality of care. There is likely to be a reduction in self-care with a significant shift towards primary care. Practices will be supporting families and those living on their own. Health care must aim to support families and neighbours in their community.

4. Economy and working conditions

Despite increasing disposable income, there is a widening gap in terms of wealth between those in the top and bottom quintile of households. Employment is shifting towards the service industries and sick-leave is high. In the future, there is likely to be a core of essential workers with a significant non-core of temporary workers. These effects will further widen inequalities in health.

5. Science and technology

Rapid advances in medicine, communications and information technology means that more can potentially be done in medicine. With improved technology, more people are likely to be cared for within the community. The effect will be higher patient expectations and with more care being provided within primary care. This will involve the primary care team in new roles, and the requirement of further training and education. There must be the careful introduction of new innovations after proper evaluation.

6. Health and social policy, patterns of service

With increasing morbidity, referrals to secondary care will increase. Unless services match demand, waiting times for secondary care services will increase. The District General Hospital will change rapidly as we move towards fewer hospitals and a few highly specialized regional units. It is likely that community care units will develop and involve the primary care team. The effect will be a further increase in workload and an increasing pool of treatable morbidity in the community requiring support from primary care. The expectations of consumers are likely to add further pressures.

7. *Disease prevalence*
The pattern for some diseases is changing and this will influence the demand for health care service. For example, with the predicted reduction in coronary heart disease in the future, there will be less demand for secondary care resources.

Changes in health care
Change is likely to continue rapidly and as a discontinuous process. Up to now change has largely been a continuous process with a gradual, predictable and step-wise development. This process is now becoming discontinuous with rapid, unpredictable and non-incremental development occurring. For those not prepared for change, the process will be quite unsettling and stressful since most people find change difficult. Those prepared for change will benefit from the many opportunities and find the process rewarding. Having the skills to handle change will be important. The rate of adoption of change varies and there are several clearly defined groups (Box 1.2).

Box 1.2
Rate of adoption of change

Innovators	2.5%
Early adopters	13.5%
Early majority	34%
Late majority	34%
Laggards	16%

There is a need to understand the process and implementation of change.

A number of changes have already taken place in the new market system. Health care purchasers and providers have become established with hospital trusts in secondary care and fund holding in primary care. Already the number of Health Authorities has been reduced by two-thirds and the proportion of the population covered by fundholding has increased to 50%. Other changes have been seen: an expansion in the out-of-hours schemes, the formation of the new Health Authorities, shared-care schemes involving primary care in an expanded role and a new complaints system. With the recent White Paper on Primary Care (1996), further change is unavoidable.

Managed care, through fundholding, has attempted to allocate funding on a health needs basis with the separation of provider and purchaser. This has been within a fixed budget and a regulated market. The idea has been that this funding is then used both efficiently and effectively to provide improved health care outcomes. In reality there has been little evaluation of fundholding and any available evidence is equivocal. The pattern of hospital referrals is similar for fundholding and non-fundholding practices (Coulter and Bradlow, 1993). Prescribing costs have shown a small reduction (6%) in fundholding compared with non-fundholding practices which has been lost after three years of fundholding. The difference was generated by lowering the average cost per item, through increased generic prescribing, rather than by giving fewer items (Harris and Scrivener, 1996). Many of the service improvements, attributed to fundholding, have been due to other health service changes, i.e. the Patients' Charter and the waiting list initiative. The operational costs of fundholding have been high at 3.5% of the total fundholding budget, with additional indirect costs. There is an urgent need for outcome studies of the different managed care models to be undertaken.

With the new Health Authorities has come the opportunity to integrate the planning and implementation of services. This integration will result in an increasingly local and participative service. The new authorities have new commissioning powers and hopefully the result will be a more flexible service and a shorter development cycle. The planned effect will be new local service agreements, provider flexibility and the focus on the specific needs of the community.

Local service agreements will allow the development of additional services that can be based in primary care. For example, chiropody and physiotherapy. Provider flexibility, owing to primary–secondary care boundaries not being physically separated, will allow the development of shared care and community care services. Many areas already have shared care schemes, mostly as specialist outreach clinics. Shared care schemes are likely to expand as care continues to shift from secondary care into primary care.

The focus on the specific needs of the community is now possible owing to the integration of planning. The previous separation meant that secondary care resources were less focused, which sometimes resulted in inappropriate services. The changing role of secondary care will also cause some specialized services to be moved into regional or tertiary centres.

The recent White Paper, Choice and Opportunity (1996), proposes removing the current contractual restraints. This will allow the extension of General Medical Services, so that new models of care delivery can be piloted. Service planning will move from a national to a local focus, and provide flexibility in the provision of services to meet the health needs and circumstances of the locality. Primary care professionals will be able to use their skills to the full, providing opportunities and incentives, to promote change. Practice team-working will need to be more effective and the traditional primary care partnership, a hierarchical model, will need to change to one of equality and task orientation.

Primary health care team

The current primary health care team has evolved in a disorganized and reactive way. It currently consists of three different teams: the core, attached and community teams. The core team consists of the general practitioners, practice manager, practice nurses and administrative staff. The attached team consists of the district nurse, health visitor, midwife, dietician, social worker and others. The community team with the stoma-care nurse, palliative-care nurse and others work in the community.

These teams often reflect the traditional boundaries that have existed between the different professional groups and levels of care. Over time some fundamental differences have developed between the core and attached teams. The core team has typically been based in general practice, been autonomous and has provided care for the local community. It is managed by the practice with most of the work being carried out within the practice. The attached team has typically been managed by secondary care, is not autonomous and is based on a geographical area with most of the work being carried out in the community.

This organizational structure has meant that team working within and between the different teams has often been ineffective. The problems have often been a power culture, with poor team vision and planning. These problems cause poor team attitudes and performance. Ultimately, patient care is affected. The recognition of ineffective team working often goes unnoticed until problems present. The symptoms, weak communication, conflict, performance issues, stress, complaints, unhappiness and loss of staff, are often present, but remain unrecognized.

> *There was an important job to be done and **everybody** was asked to do it. **Anybody** could have done it but **nobody** did it. **Somebody** got angry because it was **everybody's** job. **Everybody** thought **anybody** could do it, but **nobody** realized that **everybody** wouldn't do it. It ended up that **everybody** blamed **somebody** when actually **nobody** asked **anybody**.*

Ineffective team working results in a power culture, unclear goals, poor participation, weak interaction, unclear roles and the sense of there being no time. In the future, teams and their effective working will be an essential requirement to meet the demands facing primary care. The role and skills of different members of the team have remained largely unchanged. In the future, a fundamentally different team structure, together with new skills, will be required to overcome the current barriers to team working.

Changes are already taking place. Recently, there has been a rapid expansion of primary care nursing. Practice nursing numbers have increased by 400% over the last 10 years. However, the role and responsibilities of the practice nurse are sill constrained by regulations together with the culture and attitudes of the medical profession. Though there is still controversy around the nature and scope of their role, the number of nurse practitioners, who work independently managing their own medical problems, has expanded rapidly. In 1996, some 300 nurse practitioners had already graduated from the Royal College of Nursing's course, most to work in primary care. The demand for nurse practitioners in both primary and secondary care continues to increase. Numbers are set to rise markedly as new courses come on stream.

FUTURE STATE OF UK HEALTH CARE

The danger is that 'caring' services will know the price of everything and the value of nothing. (Welsh Health Planning Forum)

The current model of UK health care has been undergoing further review and change. It will face significant new developments in the future. The managed care market will develop further and continue to be regulated in order to maintain competition. The problem of an infinite demand for health care being met by finite resources is not new. There have always been finite resources and rationing of care but the process has now become more explicit. The process of priority setting or rationing involves medical decisions about individual patients. Decisions in the past have largely been based on purely clinical grounds involving the likely outcome of a treatment and the patient's capacity to benefit from it. Other influences such as financial and societal issues are now becoming factors in the decision-making process. It may be that priority setting has to be made on the basis of society's beliefs and ethics. Examples often attract publicity resulting in a media influence.

The market will continue to be regulated as a managed market. Regulation is required in order to prevent market failures, to provide guaranteed access to services and to support other functions such as medical research and training. Effective market management requires some core elements (Box 1.3) (Ham and Maynard, 1994).

Managed care aims at controlling costs by aggressive management of health provision and finance. Managed care consists of a variety of strategies to integrate finance and delivery of health care, and control utilization of health services and costs to improve efficiency. Health care in the UK has been managed since the beginning of the NHS and the recent reforms made contracting and purchasing more explicit.

Future principles of health care

The traditional principles of the service, availability, accessibility and accountability will be extended to include the principles of consumer choice, quality of care and value for money (Welsh Health Planning Group,1994).

Box 1.3
Core elements to
effective market
management

♦ Openness of information

♦ Control of labour and capital markets

♦ Regulation of mergers and takeovers

♦ Arbitration between purchasers and providers

♦ Protection of non-profit-making functions

♦ Overseeing provision of services

♦ Protection of basic principles of the National Health Service (NHS)

♦ Overseeing closures and redundancies

1. Consumer choice

Consumers will have choice. The users of the service should be able to exercise maximum control over their health, treatment and the care they receive. The process will involve the consumer in all areas of health care.

♦ Health and social services should support and encourage people to maintain and improve their health and well-being.
♦ Service users and carers should influence the development of services.
♦ All users should have equal access to the best available care.
♦ People should have access to appropriate information to enable them to make real choices about the care they receive.
♦ Whenever appropriate and acceptable to people, services should be provided in the home, near the home or in a homely setting.

2. Quality of care

Quality of care will be increasingly important and will be judged from the point of view of the person using the service. The result will be a move towards patient-centred outcomes. Quality indicators will be required both for the practice and for the practitioners. Both the consumer and managers as part of a quality assurance process will use these indicators.

♦ Services should strive to provide the most effective treatment and care possible.
♦ Care should be geared to the user's needs and not organizational convenience.
♦ Staff should be responsive to users and carers.

3. Value for money

The maximum possible benefit should be extracted from every pound spent.

◆ The investment must be in what is effective in meeting the needs of the users and clients, and in what they value.

◆ Everyone entrusted with resources should ensure that services are managed cost effectively.

◆ Staff should be able to use their skills to the full, while making sure that service users receive the appropriate level of expertise at every stage.

◆ Day-to-day management control should be devolved as close as possible to where care is given.

Key trends for the future

Several key trends can be identified.

1. Lifelong health

There will be an increasing focus on health, its maintenance and the prevention of ill-health. The consumer will become increasingly informed about health and the impact of the environment. People will become more responsible for their own health care. Practices will need to collect data on their population's health status. This will require the effective use of information technology and new epidemiological skills to carry out this extended public health role.

2. Holistic care

Health and social needs will be met by locally based care services within primary care, which will require the integration of health and social care at the primary care level. Services would be provided locally to meet the consumer's needs and appear as seamless care, where the consumer would not be aware of the different agencies involved.

3. Relocation of specialist care and support

Hospital-based care will move into the community and secondary care will increasingly provide specialist care. Tertiary centres are likely to become superspecialist regional units and some will merge into secondary care units. It is likely that secondary care will have fewer centres with the further amalgamation of secondary care units. This will result in each secondary care unit caring for a population of 1–2 million rather than 250 000 as at present.

There are a number of reasons for this shift towards primary care. Patients are less likely to receive inpatient care and when they do, face a shorter inpatient time. Day care has increased with many procedures now carried out in secondary care, day-care units. In the future it is estimated that eventually 60% of procedures will be carried out as day-care procedures. Shared care has expanded through 'hospital-at-home' schemes and outreach clinics, where outpatient services are provided in primary care. Technology has improved with the result that more diagnostic and management procedures can be carried out in primary care. Primary care teams have expanded into multidisciplinary units that support and provide some secondary care services, supported by guideline developments. The result is that general practice will be expected to deliver more, higher quality of care. New clinical skills will be required with some degree of specialization amongst primary health care professionals.

4. Patterns of care

There will be a greater diversity in the patterns of care. The local involvement of the consumer and the freedom for local initiatives to develop will result in services adapting to meet the needs of a local population. This will result in a wide diversity in the patterns of care and will involve several different health care groups working together in a number of different ways. The delivery of care will be closer to where patients live and be more integrated within the local community.

5. Funding

Governments will continue to control costs and at the same time continue to ensure access and quality of the services. The European Community's role in health care will increase, which may cause problems for the UK. It is likely that private funding will increase if health care expenditure is to be maintained at the current low levels of the proportion of GDP or to be increased. The proportion of GDP spent on health care can be kept down by a strong primary care filter. A poor filter results in higher secondary care utilization. In the future, further resources will be required to support primary care's extended role.

Even within primary care the distribution of resources is unequal and is based on historical patterns of distribution. In secondary care, distribution has been controlled for the last 25 years by the resource allocation formula, which is based on weighted capitation. If this formula was applied to primary care, then there would be a significant redistribution of resources. For example, funding for the South West would be reduced by 15%, from £405m to £348m, and increased by 10% in the North, from £358m to £392m. It is likely that some redistribution will occur.

6. Labour market

General practitioners are facing a major recruitment problem. Whilst numbers have increased over the last 10 years by 10%, it is worrying that the number of training registrars has reduced by 15%. In many areas there are few GP registrars entering training and the signs are that this will rapidly become worse. Over the next 5 years, more GPs will retire than usual, 15% of the workforce, particularly as many of those recruited from overseas in the 1960s are due to leave the profession. Recruitment has not been helped by the high stress levels and low morale present in general practice.

The shortage of general practitioners has highlighted further the issue of substitution. Other health care professionals could do some of the traditional work carried out by general practitioners, i.e. nurses and pharmacists. This skill mix would mean a change in the contractual process from the individual to a team contract. As substitution occurs it is likely that average list sizes will increase from the current 1900 patients per whole-time general practitioner. Substitution would help solve some of the problems created by poor recruitment to general practice and the redistribution of resources.

7. Substitution

Skill mix is the balance between trained and untrained, qualified and unqualified, and supervisory and operative staff, within a service as well as between different staff groups (Medical Workforce Standing Advisory Committee, 1995). Already there are initiatives to review the traditional boundaries of competence between the various health professional groups. Inter-professional skill mix is increasingly being developed in order to facilitate the transfer of tasks across traditional professional boundaries. In nursing, advanced nursing roles have developed with the physician assistant, clinical nurse practitioner and nurse practitioner. It is the nurse practitioner role that has the potential to be involved in primary care skill mix. The nurse practitioner, working within a defined remit, is able to manage a caseload and see patients independently, for medical problems. Examples include diabetic clinics, health promotion programmes and acute minor illnesses. The development of multidisciplinary team working is being facilitated with the use of agreed protocols between the professional groups.

Future models of health care The current market system with the purchaser–provider split is likely to be retained. This system will continue to be regulated in order to allow competition, guarantee continued access to services and support other areas such as research and training. Regulation will bring changes to allow further competition from other health care providers, such as the private sector.

Funding of primary care will become based on a resource allocation formula that has, so far, not been applied to primary care. This will result in a significant redistribution in funding for some areas of the country.

Primary care contracts will change to allow more flexibility in the provision of services. The current contract between the individual doctor and the Health Authority will continue, but two new options will develop. These are a primary care team contract and a salaried service. With the team contract, the team would contract with the Health Authority to provide services at an agreed standard and cost. The team would be responsible for the health care of a local population. This type of contract would be the natural progression of the fund-holding model. The salaried contract would mean the doctor being an employee, which is increasingly attractive for some doctors. Other models proposed involve a fundamental change in the current purchaser–provider model (Health Policy and Economic Research Unit, 1995).

The current purchaser–provider separation is likely to be retained, with a mixture of fund-holding and commissioning models. One of the problems for purchasers has been basing their decisions on the health needs of the population rather than individuals. In the future, needs assessment tools will become refined and applied to the purchaser decision process.

The move to base secondary care services in primary care and the development of multidisciplinary teams will result in the provision of a broader range of services.

Structure of health care

The likely structure of the health care system to meet these changes will involve community care units and high-technology specialist centres (Health Policy and Economic Research Unit, 1994b). The District General Hospital as we know it today will no longer exist. It is anticipated that there will be 25–40 high-technology, and trauma and emergency centres, each serving a population of 1–2 million. Services provided from these centres will concentrate on trauma and emergency, radiotherapy, oncology, neurosciences, high-technology medicine and surgery, complex maternity, paediatric, and gynaecology services.

The primary care units will bring together primary, community and social care. These units will include a number of health care professionals as an expanded team. Services provided from these units will be a wide range of low-technology medicine and surgery, together with investigations, such as ultrasound, pathology, etc. Additional services will include supporting acute care at home and providing a minor injury service.

Primary health care team

The process of implementing the anticipated changes in health care will require a different type of primary health care team, which will be very different from the team that we have today. Other members of the team will take up some of the traditional roles of doctors. There will need to be a change in the structure of the primary health care team from a hierarchical to a task-orientated structure. Doctors have dominated the traditional hierarchical structure. The result has often been a single vision, team centred on the individuals, low motivation and team stagnation. With a task-orientated structure, the team works together to develop a strategy and a plan for its implementation. The result is a shared vision, the job rather than the person being central, and a high level of motivation and innovation.

The key to success is the people, as they are the most valuable assets in any organization. It will be people that will become increasingly valuable and important assets of the team. It will be the humanistic rather than the organizational skills that will be the key to effective team working. An ideal team will need to be proactive, productive and personal. For effective team working the individual will need to feel important to the team, perform tasks that are meaningful and rewarding, and have their contributions identified and evaluated. The team itself will need the tasks to be interesting to perform and to have clear goals. There will need to be feedback on the team member's performance. The benefits to the team will be enormous. There will be: sharing of problems, improved business relationships, sharing of skills and knowledge, problem solving, enhanced motivation, and a good team spirit. The effect will be effective and coordinated care and ultimately improved quality of care for the patient. In the long-term it will be these highly motivated primary care teams that will have a competitive advantage over other less efficient and effective teams. It is likely that, as the market develops, so there will be the development of preferred provider status in primary care.

The improved competitive advantage and the strong business viability of these primary care units make it likely that the weaker businesses will not survive. It will be vital that in the future practices are managed effectively.

Disadvantages to health care   While many of the changes will result in an improved service for the consumer, there are a number of potential disadvantages. These include loss of practice individuality, loss of personal care, changes in advocacy and changes in professional power.

1. Practice individuality
The loss of practice individuality may result from the move towards larger primary care units or collaboration between practices. For many people, the individuality of care has been a special feature of general practice. This individuality has often been associated with innovation.

2. Personal care
The involvement of an increasing number of people in care will result in the loss of continuous and personal care. Responsibility is shared and the consumer will be faced with a number of carers. It is interesting that one of the key values for patients has been personal care and the loss of this will be seen as one of the major disadvantages of the changes. The move towards out-of-hours schemes has been part of this.

3. Advocacy

The changing role of the health care individual will affect advocacy. Traditionally, the carer has been the patient's advocate with decisions based on the patient's interests rather than those of the health professional. With the development of managed care and rationing it is likely that advocacy will change. This will present some difficult ethical decisions in the future.

4. Professional power

For doctors, the move towards a task-orientated team and the delegation of roles to other groups will result in a loss of professional power. For many, the sharing of power will require a fundamental change in attitudes and culture, which are often the main barriers to change.

IMPLICATIONS FOR PRIMARY CARE

Primary care units will be very different in the future. General practitioners will need additional skills in order to take up the new roles. The management areas are particularly important, as many of the skills required are new to the practitioners. Effective management skills will facilitate the securing of limited resources and the provision of a high quality of care and a competitive advantage in the market.

Clinical

Even in the area of traditional clinical skills, there will need to be change. A higher quality of clinical care is necessary for practices to be able to deliver a high-quality, extended range of care. Most will require the skills to provide a basic level of clinical care but will need, in addition, some specialization in specific clinical area.

Managed care

The principle of managed care is being established in many countries to contain costs. This creates a dilemma between the managers, who want value for money, and the doctors who want health care at any cost. Understanding the principles, processes and outcomes of managed care will be important in securing resources and guaranteeing their efficient use (see Chapter 2).

Practice objectives, planning and strategy

With the move towards primary-care-led health care, practices are becoming more independent and business orientated. General practice, as a business, will require planning skills. This will involve the development of business plans, with a vision for the future, and statements of practice objectives with strategies for their implementation (Chapter 4).

Ethics of health care

There will always be ethical dilemmas in practice and the rate of occurrence of these situations is increasing. The specific areas that are important to our practice are confidentiality, teamwork, limited resources, advocacy, professional boundaries and medical advances. Awareness of potential ethical dilemmas and having the skills of moral reasoning are important for a doctor to be effective. Furthermore, the nature, origins and effects of an ethical dilemma need to be understood together with the development of the skills to manage such a moral dilemma (Chapter 3).

Negotiation

Sound negotiation skills are required in a number of areas. In the purchaser–provider market of managed care, contracts and service provision have to be negotiated. In particular there is a need for more effective skills in contract management, which can then maximize the chances of a satisfactory outcome. Both the team and the individual can benefit from the use of negotiation skills. The degree of success that the process of negotiation achieves in securing resources will have a direct impact on patient care (Chapter 5).

Team management

There will be an increased need for team working. The delivery of primary care will be through teams. The benefits of a multidisciplinary approach need to be understood. The skills required include an understanding of the evolving models of the team approach to management in primary care, the identification of the different roles within the team and the dynamic processes involved. Furthermore, the barriers to effective teamworking need to be understood and recognized (Chapter 6).

Statutory and legal responsibilities

Practitioners will be required to work within a more stringent legal framework. The legal issues include partnership law, confidentiality, negligence and complaints. Employers have medical and non-medical responsibilities. These responsibilities include duty of care, health and safety, employment law, national statutory requirements and contractual issues. The whole area is rapidly changing, particularly with the influence of the European Union (Chapter 7).

Financial management

The contractual changes to general practice have resulted in additional effort to increase incomes, reduce expenses and to maintain profitability as an independent business. Practices need to control and manage their financial resources effectively. Financial management will become essential for practices to survive. As a result, an understanding of the tools used are important. These include the principles of budgeting and forecasting, the use of a balance sheet together with profit and loss accounts, and the role of the annual practice accounts. In addition, financial monitoring, together with key financial indicators of practice performance, are required for effective financial planning (Chapter 8).

Technological management

The demands for information audits in general practice are increasing all the time. Information technology (IT) systems need to be effective in the administration of routine tasks, maintenance of the clinical record, and need to have the ability to audit and extract data. However, for many practices, the use of IT is patchy and ineffective. This is unfortunate as the appropriate use of IT can make a significant contribution to the practice. Practices need to understand clearly what can be achieved with the effective use of IT and the implications for the future (Chapter 9).

Management of people

The management of people is the most important aspect of management in practice. The process starts with the business plan together with an assessment of people's competencies required to implement the plan. Recruitment and performance monitoring follow this. The effective handling of performance and discipline problems within a legal framework require particular skills. It is the interpersonal skills that are crucial for success and are essential for those in a management role (Chapter 10).

CONCLUSION The changes in health care have large implications for primary care. As managed care is established, so health care professionals will become increasingly accountable to both management and consumers. Change will continue rapidly and as a discontinuous process. For those not prepared for change, the process will be quite unsettling and stressful. Those prepared for change will benefit from the many opportunities and find the process rewarding.

The process of implementing the anticipated changes in health care will require a different type of primary health care team, which will be very different to the team that we have today. The key to success is the people, as they are the most valuable assets in any organization. It will be people that will become increasingly valuable and important assets of the team. General practitioners will need additional skills in order to take up new roles. The management areas are particularly important, as many of the skills required are new to the practitioners.

It will be those practices who are managed effectively that will have a competitive advantage in the evolving managed care market.

SUMMARY

◆ Western health care systems are going through a time of rapid change and these changes will affect all those involved in providing health care.

◆ Primary care will need to be able to adapt to the process of continual change and to make effective use of resources.

◆ The traditional principles of the service, availability, accessibility and accountability will be extended to include the principles of consumer choice, quality of care and value for money.

◆ The process of implementing the anticipated changes in health care will require a different type of primary health care team, which will be very different to the team that we have today.

◆ The key to success is the people, as they are the most valuable assets in any organization. It will be people that will become increasingly valuable and important assets of the team.

FURTHER READING

◆ Health Care UK (1995/96), *An Annual Review of Health Care Policy.* King's Fund, London.

A good overall review of health care changes in the UK. In addition, there are some analysis chapters looking at some of the specific issues.

◆ Health Policy and Economics Research Unit, *Discussion Papers.* BMA, London.

An excellent ongoing series on key issues and dilemmas. Each discussion paper carefully assesses the issue, the possible solutions and their likely impact.

◆ *UK Health Care: The Facts.* Orton, P. and Fry, J. (1995) Kluwer Academic Publishers, Lancaster.

This book is a rich source of information on the UK system, selecting, interpreting and putting into context the vast amount of information. Sets the issues in their context.

◆ *Future Options for General Practice.* Edited by Geoff Meads (1996) Radcliffe Medical Press, Oxford.

A good overall view of the options facing primary care together with examples of schemes that have been implemented.

◆ *The Nature of General Medical Practice* (1996) Royal College of General Practitioners, London.

A good overview of the disciplines and skills that general practitioners will require in the future. The implications for clinical competence are considered.

REFERENCES

Choice and Opportunity. White Paper 1996. London: HMSO.

Coulter, A. and Bradlow, J. (1993), Effect of NHS reforms on general practitioners' referrals. *British Medical Journal* **306**: 433-6.

Ham, C. and Maynard, A. (1994), Core elements of effective market management. Managing the NHS market. *British Medical Journal* (6932) 308.

Harris, C. and Scrivener, G. (1996) Fundholders' prescribing costs: the first five years. *British Medical Journal* 313: 1531-4.

Health Policy and Economic Research Unit (1994a), *Accountability in the NHS: A Discussion Paper.* December, London: BMA.

Health Policy and Economic Research Unit (1994b), *Future Models of Healthcare.* June. London: BMA.

Health Policy and Economic Research Unit (1995), *Future Models for the NHS: A Discussion Paper.* April. London: BMA.

Medical Workforce Standing Advisory Committee (1995), *Planning the Medical Workforce.* Second Report, June. London: DOH.

Welsh Health Planning Group (1994), *Health and Social Care 2010: A Report on Phase One.* April.

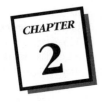

MANAGED CARE: CROSSING THE ATLANTIC

CHAPTER 2

Alan Maynard and Karen Bloor

OBJECTIVES

- ♦ To explore the role of managed care in the context of the goals of health care systems and health reforms.

- ♦ To show the different models and components of a managed care system.

- ♦ To make comparisons between managed care in the USA and UK.

- ♦ To evaluate the outcomes of managed care and its role in the future of the National Health Service.

INTRODUCTION

Managed care 'marches inexorably forward' as 'the solution' to causes of expenditure inflation in the USA (Hiebert-White, 1995). Interest in the concept has crossed the Atlantic. This chapter considers managed care in the context of the goals of health care systems and health reforms. The first section focuses on the objectives of the British National Health Service (NHS): will managed care facilitate or frustrate the achievement of these goals? The second section examines managed care in both USA and UK contexts, giving examples of the different models of managed care. The third section evaluates managed care in the USA: the various systems in place, evidence of their advantages and disadvantages, and overall impact on health care expenditure and outcomes. The final section considers which constituents of managed care may be applicable to the British NHS in general, and primary care in particular.

HEALTH CARE SYSTEM OBJECTIVES

During the last decade, policy makers in a large number of countries including the UK have attempted various reforms of their health care systems, indeed health care reform has been described as a 'global epidemic' (Klein, 1993). All such reforms consist of very complex policy choices, but policy makers are often reluctant to define their objectives, as clarity about what they are seeking to achieve may enhance their accountability and the political distress caused when policy targets are not achieved. There are three important targets in all health care systems (Maynard and Bloor, 1995) (Box 2.1).

Box 2.1
Health care system
targets

- ◆ Cost control
- ◆ Efficiency
- ◆ Equity

Macroeconomic cost control   Spending limits are necessary because the combined effects of private market failure and government policy lead to both excess demand and excess supply of health services. In a private market, uncertainty about future health and future need for health care leads individuals to take out medical insurance. This means that once insured, patients are not responsible for paying for their treatment – a third party (the insurer) pays. In a government-funded system, the effect is the same: neither patients nor the doctors treating them have any incentive to use resources economically. Consequently, costs and expenditure inflate. This inflation is exacerbated by a fee for service remuneration system, where providers' income is increased by the provision of more diagnostic and therapeutic interventions. Increased health care expenditure always and everywhere increases the incomes of health care providers. Such factors lead to the rate of growth of health care expenditure exceeding the inflation rate in many countries. For example, in the US health care system, cost inflation has led to over 14% of the US gross domestic product (GDP) being spent annually on health care ($1000 billion). The Congressional Budget Office (1994) estimated that this would rise to 20% of GDP without the Clinton health care reform plan, and 19% with it. With or without reform it is likely that one in five American dollars will be spent on health care in the early years of the next millennium. A publicly financed system faces similar inflationary pressures, although these can be ameliorated by using capitation or salaried remuneration systems, a primary care gatekeeper, and controlling expenditure with cash limits (a cap) and a single source of finance, usually taxation, which is easier to control than fragmented multiple sources of funding.

In both public and private systems, health care expenditure is a matter of policy concern for government. In publicly financed systems, the government's desire to limit public expenditure of all government departments, including health, means that cost control is a primary policy goal. In private health care systems, costs tend to fall on employers, which affects wage bills. In recent years in the USA, there have been relatively small increases in wages, and rewards have largely consisted of benefits in kind, of which health care is a primary element. The increasing costs of health insurance are significant costs to employers which affect international competitiveness of firms. This is a policy concern in the USA and in other countries, such as France and Germany, which rely on payroll taxes. The control of expenditure growth in health care systems is a policy goal which dominates the behaviour of governments worldwide.

Microeconomic efficiency

Enhancements in the length and quality of life should be produced at minimum cost by balanced investments in health care and other determinants of health (e.g. income redistribution, education and housing). Efficiency goals require the identification of structural arrangements (e.g. technology assessment), which increase the productivity of the health sector.

The identification of efficiency requires both the determination of the cost effectiveness of competing interventions (technical efficiency) and the preferences of society (allocative efficiency).

If societies (and the governments which represent them) wish to allocate access to health care, not on the basis of willingness and ability to pay, as in private markets, but in relation to need, it is necessary to allocate health care resources by the capacity of patients to benefit from care. Meeting this allocation principle efficiently means allocating by capacity to benefit per unit of cost. Policy makers and resource allocators have to make two judgements, if their actions are directed by the benefit principle. Such governments must:

♦ Identify which treatments are cost effective, as only then can they target scarce resources to maximize 'health gains' from the health care budget. This requires identification of effectiveness (evidence based medicine) and this to be linked with cost, i.e. how much patient health status is improved by a unit of investment.

♦ Decide how much they will pay from public expenditure to buy additional health gains (e.g. quality adjusted life-years).

The pursuit of an efficiency goal requires systematic technology assessment and the rapid application of new research knowledge in terms of changes in clinical practice. Generally these processes, research and development, are inadequate, and the task of eroding existing inefficiencies is difficult.

Equity

The results of economic evaluation (the identification of resource costs and patient effectiveness) inform public choices. The eventual decision about who will be treated, and who will not, should reflect both this information and social values, which means that efficiency goals can be over-ridden by equity considerations. As Fuchs (1974, p. 148) argued:

> *At the root of most of our major health problems are value choices. What kind of people are we? What kind of life do we want to lead? What kind of society do we want to build for our children and grandchildren? How much weight do we want to put on individual freedom? How much to equality? How much to material progress? How much to the realm of the spirit? How important is our own health to us? How important is our neighbour's health to us? The answers we give to these questions, as well as the guidance we get from economics, will and should shape health care policy.*

Thus it may be technically inefficient for society to keep alive very low birthweight babies (e.g. <500 g) because of the high incidence of physical and intellectual disability. However, societies may decide that letting neonates die prematurely is unacceptable and that the health care system should deliver care which is inefficient in terms of cost effectiveness but desired by society. The principles behind such choices should be identified clearly to facilitate accountability. They may reflect values such as a belief that citizens should have a 'fair innings', i.e. an expectation of, say, 70 years of good quality life. After a 'fair innings' citizens should reasonably expect that the NHS will not 'strive officiously' (and inefficiently) to keep people alive.

US health care objectives

Policy makers in health care systems accord different rankings to these three fundamental objectives. For example, the US health care system has historically been structured to create cost inflation and policy makers have tended to argue that efficiency will create cost containment. US policy makers also give little attention to equity, as access to health care is determined by ability to pay. The health care system is fragmented and dominated by insurance for employees, funded by employers. Medicare and Medicaid programmes, covering elderly people, those with certain chronic diseases and some (not all) poor people mitigate partially these equity problems, but gaps in coverage remain. Around 40 million Americans are uninsured at any given time, and 50-60 million may be without insurance at some time during a calendar year (Schroeder, 1996).

The dominance of the interests of the insured population in the US health care policy debate, owing to cost inflation and its perceived deleterious effect on international competitiveness, has generated reform aimed at controlling costs by aggressive micromanagement of health provision and finance (managed care) (Box 2.2).

Box 2.2
Managed care

Aims to control costs by aggressive micromanagement of health provision and finance.

UK health care objectives   The UK health care system has, since the inception of the NHS, given priority to equity issues, enabling universal access to health care, and to cost containment, with a single pipe of tax finance and central control of salary levels. Prior to the 1991 reforms, the NHS 'would appear to have been the most highly centralized health care system in the OECD area' (Organisation for Economic Co-operation and Development (OECD), 1994). The majority of funding continues to be derived from taxes: direct taxation (82%), payroll levies (13%), and 4% from user charges (Department of Health, 1994).

This centralized structure has maintained relative cost control: in 1992 the UK spent 7.1% of its GDP on health care, compared to an average of 9.9% in the OECD as a whole and 13.8% in the USA (Office of Health Economics, 1995) (Figure 2.1). Outcomes, in terms of health status, appear to be comparable with those achieved in other countries, making the NHS 'a remarkably cost-effective institution' (OECD, 1994). The pre-1991 NHS had a number of advantages, including universal coverage and cost control. However, the incentives for efficiency in service provision were muted or even perverse. For example, if hospitals treated more patients by exploiting new technologies, they were likely to exhaust their fixed annual budgets prematurely and reduce activity. Also, with cash-limited hospital budgets and demand-determined primary care budgets there was an incentive to shift patients and

Figure 2.1
Total health expenditure as a percentage of GDP at market prices in selected OECD countries, 1992.

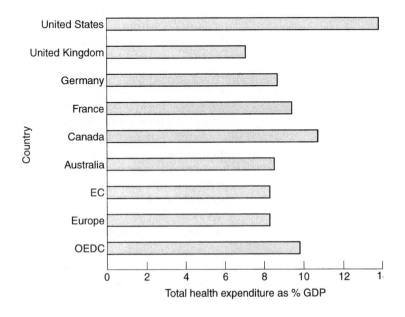

Total health expenditure as % GDP

costs from one sector to another regardless of efficiency. The 1991 reforms, with an 'internal market' and aspects of US-style managed competition, aimed to increase incentives for efficiency. Cost containment and access (equity) policies remained unchanged, with continued funding primarily from direct taxation.

WHAT IS MANAGED CARE? The term 'managed care' is used often, interpreted widely, and can be used to describe a variety of different models of health care finance and delivery. It is defined by Iglehart (1994) as:

> *... a system that, in varying degrees, integrates the financing and delivery of medical care through contracts with selected physicians and hospitals that provide comprehensive health care services to enrolled members for a predetermined monthly premium. All forms of managed care represent attempts to control costs by modifying the behaviour of doctors, although they do so in different ways.*

Managed care, therefore, represents a variety of strategies to control utilization of health services and costs, and may be viewed as resembling the pre-reform NHS in terms of integrating finance and delivery of care. It is remarkable that this US 'innovation' is the opposite of UK policies of the early 1990s. Managed care has some core characteristics (Box 2.3).

Box 2.3
Managed care characteristics

Aggressive micromanagement of resources by:

♦ Integrating finance and delivery of health care.

♦ Modifying the behaviour of doctors.

♦ Restricting patients' choice of providers.

Managed care in the USA Managed care is not a new concept. Kaiser-Permanante, the best known health maintenance organization, was formed in California in 1942, and the roots of managed care can be traced to the funeral and benevolent societies that immigrants set up to cover death expenses in the 1800s (Friedman, 1996). A number of different organizational forms of managed care exist in the USA, including health maintenance organizations (HMO), preferred provider organizations (PPO), independent practice associations (IPA) and point of service plans (POS). Box 2.4 gives definitions of six US organizational forms of health care delivery, listed by intensity of management from least managed (traditional fee for service indemnity insurance plans) to most managed (HMO).

In 1993, 49% of employees with health insurance in the USA were enrolled in traditional indemnity insurance plans and 51% in

Box 2.4
Definitions of six
representative
organizational forms of
health care delivery
listed by intensity of
management

Organizational form*	Definition
Indemnity plan with fee for service	Complete freedom of choice to patients. Insurer reimburses physicians on a fee-for-service basis.
Managed indemnity plan	Free choice and fee for service, but insurer exercises some degree of utilization control to manage costs.
Preferred provider organization	Insurer channels patients to 'preferred' physicians who are usually paid a discounted fee for service. The insurer, not the physician, usually accepts financial risk for performance.
Independent practice association	Insurer channels patients to physicians usually solo or in small groups who have agreed to some financial risk for performance. Payment may be either capitation or fee for service with financial incentives based on performance.
Network independent practice association	Similar to independent practice association but consists of a network of larger group practices. Payment is usually capitation to each group, which then pays the physicians.
Staff/group health maintenance organization	The classic, prepaid, large multispecialt group practice. Patients are covered only for care delivered by the health maintenance organization. The physicians are usually salaried and work either for the plan (staff-model health maintenance organization) or for a physician group practice (group-model health maintenance organization) that has an exclusive contract with the plan.

*Not shown are hybrid arrangements such as open-ended and point-of-service arrangements whereby in a preferred provider organization, independent practice association, or staff/group health maintenance organizations may have some insurance coverage for care outside the providers approved by the insurer.

Source: Rivo, M.L., Mays, H.L., Katzoff, J. and Kindig, D.A. (1995), Managed care: implications for the physician workforce and education. *Journal of American Medical Association* **273**: 330–335.

managed care plans (Friedman, 1996). The largest percentage of enrolees in managed care plans were with HMOs (22%). HMOs require patients to use participating physicians for all medical care except emergencies, and physicians may be directly employed by the HMO (staff model HMO) or function in private practices contracting with the HMO (group model) (Friedman, 1996). HMOs integrate the insurance and provision functions in health care delivery, in contrast to traditional insurers, who are responsible only for reimbursing providers for services that patients have sought on their own. An HMO provides comprehensive health care for a prepaid premium, and therefore agrees to bear substantial financial risk. Individuals know better than HMOs or insurers their own health risks, and are likely to conceal relevant information where possible in order to reduce premiums. No HMO is able to predict an individual's future need for health care accurately, and a small group of individuals who develop conditions which are very expensive to treat can have a significant impact on the organization's budget. This creates incentives for reducing excessive utilization and minimizing other inefficiencies, and providing preventive care when it is cost effective (Folland *et al.*, 1993). HMOs and other managed care organizations also use a system of 'pre-certification' whereby any non-emergency hospitalization requires prior authorization to verify a doctor's recommendation.

PPOs enrolled 20% of employees with health insurance in 1993. A PPO is an arrangement under which patients are given financial incentives to receive care from a limited number of doctors and hospitals, with which the payer has contracted (Friedman, 1996). Networks of individual doctors, medical groups and hospitals contract with a plan for a discounted rate of payment. In return, plans deliver large volumes of services by giving patients a list of preferred providers. Patients can consult non-participating physicians, but pay higher out of pocket costs when they do so (Friedman, 1996). IPAs consist of solo, small groups or larger networks of practitioners who agree to some financial risk of performance and insurers channel patients to them. Payment is generally based on capitation but with some financial incentives based on performance. Finally, point of service plans, the newest (and fastest growing) form of managed care which attracted 9% of employees with insurance in 1993, represent a hybrid between more restrictive HMOs and less restrictive PPOs. PPOs plans rely on a patient selecting a physician gatekeeper, who is responsible for coordinating all medical care. Again, for an additional fee, patients can consult non-participating doctors.

Managed care in the USA, therefore, consists of aggressive micromanagement of resources by integrating finance and delivery of health care (usually by contracting), modifying doctors' behaviour and restricting patients' choice of providers. There is more emphasis on primary care and patients increasingly tend to access secondary care via primary care gatekeepers, who may be networks of nurse practitioners and primary care physicians. Access to specialists is restricted by these gatekeepers, in order to reduce the demand for specialist physicians and hospital care.

Finance of health care under a managed care plan is usually capitation based, with a prepaid premium, contrasting with a traditional fee for service remuneration. This reduces incentives for overtreatment and supplier-induced interventions. There are considerable pressures on provider organizations to reduce costs, and health plans make more profit when physicians provide less care, a reversal of the previous system of incentives. Non-emergency hospitalization often requires prior authorization (pre-certification) through a gatekeeper system. There are considerable concerns within the American medical profession that such incentives are dangerously restricting, and threaten the quality of patient care, particularly as increasing numbers of health plans are commercial enterprises rather than not-for-profit organizations.

Managed care organizations work energetically to reduce variations in practice, which are increasingly viewed as unacceptable by US clinicians. In the USA and world-wide, many clinical choices are ill-informed and made under great uncertainty and, as a consequence, there are large variations in how clinicians treat patients of similar age, sex and other characteristics (Andersen and Mooney, 1990). For example, a study of 30 hospital markets in Maine demonstrated up to eight-fold variations in surgical and medical practice (Wennburg *et al.*, 1987). Medical practice variations also exist between countries. McPherson *et al.* (1982) compared the incidence of seven common surgical procedures in England, Norway and the USA, and found that English and Norwegian rates were lower than the USA for all procedures except appendicectomy. Hysterectomy and tonsillectomy were four times as common in the USA as in Norway, prostatectomy was twice as common in the USA as in England.

Attempts to reduce variations in practice centre around development and dissemination of guidelines. Federally funded organizations such as the Agency for Health Care Policy and Research have developed a number of detailed evidence-based guidelines, which are increasingly implemented by managed care organizations. The American Medical Association now has over 1800 practice guidelines available. Clinicians in managed care organizations have much less discretion around the use of guidelines than other US (and UK) clinicians: they require adherence to guidelines and can refuse to pay and drop clinicians from their plans if guidelines are ignored. In the UK, guidelines are produced by researchers such as those in the NHS Centre for Reviews and Dissemination, but these are rarely actively implemented or monitored at a local level.

Managed care in the UK   Since the creation of the NHS, health care in the UK has been 'managed'. The UK health care system, both public and private sectors, already contains many of the components of US-style managed care. Financing and delivery of health care are integrated in that the public sector funds and provides most health care. Hospital specialists are paid by the NHS on a salary basis, and this prevents the incentives to overtreat which were present in the US system of indemnity insurance and fee-for-service reimbursement.

General practitioners (GPs) are paid largely by capitation, like HMO primary care physicians, although with some fee-for-service elements. There has always been an emphasis on primary care, and GPs treat 90% of all contacts with the health care system, and act as gatekeepers to secondary care. Patients have restricted choice of hospital specialists and, realistically, of GPs, but can, by paying directly or taking out health insurance, expand their choice of providers.

The 1991 reforms added to some of the parallels between the organization of the NHS and US-style managed care systems. Private insurance companies in the UK are also moving towards a managed care approach.

1. The purchaser–provider split
Elements of the purchaser–provider split appear to be moving away from rather than towards a US managed care system. Managed care consists of the integration of finance and delivery of care, whereas the internal market explicitly separates the two. However, the way contracting and purchasing operates in practice has parallels with US managed care. The present separation of these functions may be a necessary but temporary prerequisite to creating a more effectively managed health care system in which integrated packages of care with explicit practice guidelines are the norm.

The primary public purchasers of health services are District Health Authorities (DHAs), which cover geographically defined populations of over 300 000. They assess health needs and contract for health services, either on a block or cost per case basis, from public and private providers. These are tasks required of US managed care organizations, but without, as yet, the integration of finance and delivery of care. DHAs are, however, funded by a prepaid weighted capitation and, therefore, have incentives to take a population view of health care, and consider costs as well as effectiveness when deciding priorities. DHAs contract with certain Trusts (similar to a preferred provider list) and require extra-contractual referrals (prior authorization very similar to the US pre-certification system) for patients to be treated outside those contracts. As yet their vigour of contracting, compared to the USA, is modest but the potential for emulation is considerable and likely to be exploited increasingly particularly if NHS funding is, as it should be, parsimonious.

2. GP fundholding and total fundholding
General practice fundholding appears to have been something of an 'add-on' to the 1989 White Paper (Department of Health and Social Security, 1989), derived from academic discussions in the early 1980s (Marinker, 1984; Maynard, 1986; Maynard *et al.*, 1986). These academic discussions drew from ideas within health main-

tenance organizations in the USA, and advocated the implementation of a similar system of incentives. The fundholding scheme, as outlined in the White Paper, initially allowed general practices with patient lists exceeding 11 000 to apply for their own budgets to purchase a limited list of hospital services, including outpatient services, diagnostic tests and some non-emergency inpatient and day case treatment. The budgets also included all the primary care services provided by GPs. A minimum list size was included to reduce the risk involved with practice fundholding and if the annual cost to the practice of hospital treatment for a patient exceeded £5000 (now £6000), the excess was funded by the DHA. Subsequently, the minimum list size has been reduced to 5000 and the scope of the budget extended to cover nearly all elective surgery, outpatient therapy and specialist nursing services formerly provided by Trusts.

GP fundholders act both as providers of primary care and also purchasers of services on behalf of their practice populations, integrating finance and delivery of health care in a system similar to a mini-HMO, but with a narrower definition of services provided. Fundholders also contract with a list of 'preferred providers', although in theory patients have more choice over the provider of specialist care as GP fundholders can move patients around local health care providers at the margin without threatening overall provision. However, fundholders have weaker incentives to control costs as there is no profit motive – fundholders cannot keep any surpluses, and can only invest them in the practice.

From April 1996 over 50 fundholding practices became 'total fundholders', purchasing all their patients' health care needs in collaboration with DHAs, including accident and emergency services, medical and psychiatric inpatient care, and maternity services, which are excluded from conventional fundholding. Total fundholding is even more similar to a HMO, with similar incentive structures and substantial risk bearing. However, the scheme also excludes the profit motive and the aggressive management of resources which profit could stimulate. Continuing this move towards managed care policies in the UK NHS may lead to franchising of primary care and requires further change in the GP contract. Some of this change is already in process, for example, new arrangements for contracting for the provision of integrated packages of secondary care with practice guidelines and within general practice have been implemented (NHS Executive, 1996). This allows for further movement of services from secondary to primary care, where this is 'more convenient for patients, cost-effective, safe and of a recognized standard' (NHSE, 1996). This move from secondary to primary care provision emulates trends in US managed care organizations.

3. Private health insurance

Private health care provision and a market for private health insurance has existed alongside the NHS since its inception. However, in recent years this market has expanded and is now around £1.5 billion, covering over 10% of the population, mostly for elective procedures. Private hospitals have a capacity of approximately 12 000 beds.

To control expenditure inflation, insurers have recently developed preferred provider relations. For instance, the British United Provident Association (BUPA), which has 45% of the private health insurance market, has entered into a preferred provider relationship with a group of 150 private hospitals, which are offering up to 20% price discounts. Such arrangements are welcome to the private hospital owners as their bed utilization rates are low. The public is being directed away from pay beds in NHS hospitals (where there is better emergency care back-up) by being offered perks if they opt for a policy where treatment is restricted to the approved private units, including credits for elderly care and dental insurance, health screening and membership of fitness clubs (Dawe, 1996). The insurers also recognize the need to reduce variations in medical practice (e.g. length of stay) and see the preferred provider relations as a way of enforcing protocols to control cost and quality.

The private sector could reduce practice variations and develop practice guidelines more rapidly than the NHS, particularly as some powerful insurers (e.g. Private Patients Plan and Norwich Union) are for-profit organizations, and the gains from greater efficiency would benefit management and shareholders directly. If they are more successful, there will be a paradox: the specialists they use will be more rigorously managed in their private sector environment than when they work in their usual NHS jobs! The scope for private sector–NHS collaboration in such areas may be considerable and mutually rewarding as a result.

EVALUATING MANAGED CARE IN THE USA

Folland *et al.* (1993) suggest seven potential advantages and disadvantages of health maintenance organizations and other managed care systems in comparison to traditional US indemnity insurance systems (Box 2.5).

Box 2.5
HMO advantages and disadvantages

1. Reduce quantity and intensity of care.
2. Substitute lower cost care for higher cost care.
3. Economies in the purchase or use of inputs.
4. Quicker to develop effective utilization review.
5. Use or adopt new technology more efficiently.
6. Encourage the use of cost-effective preventative care.
7. Administrative economies.

HMOs may reduce the quantity and intensity of care

This is a major potential cost advantage of HMOs. There is an incentive to minimize utilization and reduce length of stay in hospital and length of treatment period, rather than to provide unnecessary or marginal care. This may, however, introduce incentives to 'underprovide' care, particularly by commercial for-profit organizations and where physicians remuneration may be tied to cutting prescriptions, hospital admissions and other costs. This may be ameliorated by the competition that exists between HMOs and also be the professional ethos of medical care, but the 'morality of the marketplace' continues to create some concern within the American medical profession (Kassirer, 1995).

HMOs may substitute lower cost care for higher cost care

In particular, HMOs have incentives to use outpatient care whenever possible. A report by Kaiser Permanante showed how HMOs try to balance cost control and patient care, for example, by considering outpatient (day care) alternatives for procedures such as gallbladder surgeries, appendicectomies and mastectomies (*USA Today*, 1995). HMOs are also more likely to, for example, use generic drugs rather than branded alternatives.

HMOs may enjoy economies in the purchase or use of inputs

HMOs may be better able to make efficient use of facilities and equipment, and may enjoy economies of scale. They also have a strong incentive to improve productivity and make better use of physician and non-physician inputs, such as nurse practitioners. Managed care organizations employ fewer physicians, particularly specialists, and may further change skill mix by using other practitioners. Weiner (1994) forecasted the effects of increases in the use of managed care on the requirement for physician workforce, estimating that if 40–65% of Americans receive care from integrated managed care networks in the near future, there could be a surplus of up to 163 000 patients care physicians in the USA by the year 2000, with specialists accounting for at least 85% of this surplus. This has far-reaching implications for US health care provision. Costs may be reduced, but there are concerns that this will be achieved at the expense of reduced quality of care. In particular, doctors' incentives to remain employed may threaten their professional role as a patient advocate. If the number of physicians can be reduced without reductions in care (by, for example, changing skill mix and reducing utilization), there may be scope for some emulation in the UK.

HMOs may be quicker to develop effective utilization review

HMOs have incentives to measure performance and develop controls to monitor physicians. The number of guidelines and protocols for care in existence in the USA continues to increase rapidly, and HMOs have more incentive to implement and monitor such guidelines than the traditional fee-for-service (FFS) sector, which has incentives to increase revenues by overtreating.

HMOs may use or adopt new technology more efficiently

In particular, HMOs are more likely to require evidence of efficiency before using new technologies. This may slow the proliferation of new and expensive technologies which has been one of the major reasons for expenditure inflation in the USA and elsewhere.

HMOs may encourage the use of cost-effective preventive care

The reason for this is that it reduces subsequent use of potentially more expensive curative care. This only applies if HMOs believe that enrolees will stay as members for long enough for the plan to benefit.

HMOs may enjoy administrative economies

This may be achieved by reducing paperwork and collection costs as billing procedures are simplified, owing to integrated finance and delivery systems. However, these savings may be a 'one off'. The development of systems such as utilization review and the costs of competition in terms of marketing, contracting and profit distribution to shareholders may reduce the cost savings produced by vigorous management. In the end, the results of managed care in the USA may be merely to redistribute expenditure, i.e. to reduce payments to hospitals, doctors and pharmaceutical equipment manufacturers and transfer them to administration (marketing, contracting and information technology) and profits.

Two main questions are considered in evaluations of the managed care approach in the US:

◆ Are costs lower?
◆ Is quality of care reduced as a result?

Studies attempting to answer these questions has been reviewed by Luft (1981) and Miller and Luft (1994). The 1981 review, studying data from the second half of the 1970s, found moderate to large HMO plan differences in hospital admissions, no consistent differences in hospital length of stay and similar ambulatory physician visit use.

The Rand Health Insurance Experiment (Manning *et al.*, 1984) randomly assigned patients to different plans in a controlled experiment to minimize potential selection bias (healthier patients joining managed care plans). HMO and FFS patients were compared in groups with different coinsurance rates. Total expenditures per person were $439 for the experimental group and $609 in the free care FFS group. The reduced spending was due largely to a much lower admission rate and around 40% fewer hospital days per person.

More recent studies, reviewed by Miller and Luft (1994) showed that HMO plans continued to have lower admission rates, 1–20% shorter hospital lengths of stay, the same or more physician office visits, less use of expensive procedures and tests, and greater use of preventive services. HMO and indemnity plans provided enrolees with comparable quality of care, according to process or outcome measures. A total of 14 out of 17 observations from 16 studies showed either better or equivalent quality of care for HMO enrolees compared with FFS enrolees for a wide range of conditions, diseases and interventions. There was no evidence to support the hypothesis that prepaid group practice or staff model HMOs are more effective than IPA or network model HMOs (Gray and Schlesinger, 1996). It is remarkable that the development of HMOs and managed care has been evaluated in a relatively small number of well-conducted studies: clearly policy makers in the USA, like the UK, do not wish to be confused by facts!

Despite intuitive and empirical evidence that managed care organization should reduce costs, particularly costs of inpatient care, and steady increases in the number of Americans covered by managed care plans, overall health expenditure has not been contained and until very recently has continued to increase substantially. Public and private cost containment strategies have clearly failed to bring health expenditure down in the USA. Enthoven (1993) suggests that this is not because competition has failed, but because price competition has not yet been tried. In particular has argues that HMOs will not have effective incentives to cut cost and price unless demand for health care is price elastic (i.e. responsive to changes in price), and that policies of purchasers and government have made demand price inelastic (unresponsive).

The development of HMOs and other US managed care plans has been influenced by the HMO Act of 1973, which provided Federal support for the planning and launching of not-for-profit HMOs. Legislators believed that HMOs for profit may provide lower quality care and may not meet reformers' social goals. During the 1970s, over 200 HMOs came into existence, with fewer than 20% for profit (Gray and Schlesinger, 1996). However, over the 1980s and 1990s, halting federal grants to not-for-profit HMOs and encouraging private investment at a time of greatly increasing demand for managed care plans, and changing tax structures have resulted in a number of well-publicized conversions to for-profit status. Around 46 plans converted from 1985 to another 61 have converted since then (Gray and Schlesinger, 1996). This increased access to capital and generated wealth for insiders, particularly owing to the undervaluing of conversion prices. For example, California's Inland Health Plan was converted in 1985 to a 'fair market price' of $562 000, most of which went to charity, but the new owners sold the company one year later for $37.5 million (Gray and Schlesinger, 1996). The for-profit conversions have increased fears about 'managed care and the morality of the marketplace' (Kassirer, 1995) and ethical issues in managed care (American Medical Association's Council on Ethical and Judicial Affairs, 1995). Competition and demand for reduced costs, along with declining need for specialist physicians could introduce inappropriate incentives:

Until now, there has been little empirical evidence to indicate that managed care is inferior to fee-for-service care. In fact, our professional ethos has so far acted as a sturdy constraint. Yet the incentive to remain employed is so strong that many physicians in a capitated system may not provide all the services they should, may not always be the patient's advocate, and may be reluctant to challenge the rules governing which services are appropriate.

Guidelines have been produced by the American Medical Association's (AMA) Council on Ethical and Judicial Affairs to deal with potential conflicting loyalties as physicians in the USA are expected to balance the interests of their patients with other patients, and, owing to bonuses and fee withholds, needs of patients can conflict with physicians' financial interests (AMA, 1995). These guidelines are summarized in Box 2.6.

Increasing price competition also creates concern, owing to the potential reductions in charity care and in support for research and teaching (Schroeder, 1996):

In the new era of price competition, we will find doctors and hospitals less financially able to provide charity care. To be able to respond to the market pressure being exerted by insurance companies, managed care organisations and employers, health care providers feel they must cut costs to the bone ... Academic health centers, which currently provide two thirds of all charity care, are among the most seriously affected by the changes. They enter today's price competition with higher costs because of their teaching function, the man high-technology, specialised services they offer, and the seriously ill – and costly – patients they serve. Of all providers, they are the ones most likely to have to stop cross-subsidising care for indigent patients by charging other payers more.

In the USA, surplus revenues from clinical care provided by hospitals and professionals is needed to continue support for charity care, and for research and teaching (Rogers *et al.*, 1994). Parallels can be drawn with UK teaching hospitals, particularly in

Box 2.6
Ethical issues in
managed care

1. The duty of patient advocacy is a fundamental element of the physician–patient relationship that should not be altered by the system of health care delivery in which physicians practise. Physicians must continue to place the interests of their patients first.
2. When managed care plans place restrictions on the care that physicians in the plan may provide to their patients, the following principles should be followed:
   (a) Any broad allocation guidelines that restrict care and choices – which go beyond the cost–benefit judgements made by physicians as part of their normal professional responsibilities – should be established at a policymaking level so the individual physicians are not asked to engage in *ad hoc* bedside rationing.
   (b) Regardless of any allocation guidelines or gatekeeper directives, physicians must advocate for any care they believe will materially benefit their patients.
   (c) Physicians should be given an active role in contributing their expertise to any allocation process and should advocate for guidelines that are sensitive to differences among patients.
   (d) Adequate appellate mechanisms for both patients and physicians should be in place to address disputes regarding medically necessary care.
   (e) Managed care plans must adhere to the requirements of informed consent that patients be given full disclosure of material information.
   (f) Physicians should also continue to promote full disclosure to patients enrolled in managed care organizations.
   (g) Physicians should not participate in any plan that encourages or requires care at or below minimum professional standards.
3. When physicians are employed or reimbursed by managed care plans that offer financial incentives to limit care, costs should not place patient welfare at risk.
   (a) Any incentives to limit care must be disclosed fully to patients.
   (b) Limits should be placed on the magnitude of fee withholds, bonuses and other financial incentives to limit care. Calculating incentive patients according to the performance of a group of physicians rather than individually should be encouraged.
   (c) Health plans should develop financial incentives based on quality of care.
4. Patients have an individual responsibility to be aware of the benefits and limitations of their health care coverage. Patients should exercise their autonomy by public participation in the formulation of benefits packages and by prudent selection of health care coverage that best suits their needs.

Source: American Medical Association Council on Ethical and Judicial Affairs (1995), Ethical issues in managed care. *Journal of American Medical Association* **273**: 330–335.

London, where even with the funding supplement from the Service Increment for Teaching and Research (SIFTR), academic centres tend to have higher capital costs, different case mixes and often higher contract prices in the internal market than their non-teaching counterparts.

MANAGED CARE AND THE FUTURE OF THE NHS Managed care is a means to an end. Thus, prior to the use of such devices, it is necessary to identify and rank the objectives (or ends) which policy makers, public and private, are pursuing. The three primary objectives of health care systems are, as discussed earlier, cost containment, efficiency and equity. Managed care pro-grammes in the USA have been used to control costs by modifying the behaviour of doctors and other providers. Managed care organization may also improve efficiency, by reducing incentives for overuse of health care resources. However, the effect on equity objectives may even be detrimental. Managed care and increased competition for providers may drive fees down, and thus reduce potential for cross-subsidization to charitable care. Managed care programmes are an alternative to traditional insurance for some employers, but may reduce access to care for the uninsured.

Before managed care type initiatives are implemented to improve efficiency in the UK NHS, it is necessary to devise a 'level playing field' in terms of equitable distribution of health care resources.

The NHS budget is decided for each of the four countries of the United Kingdom by Cabinet. The Department of Health in England (and its counterparts in Scotland, Wales and Northern Ireland) allocate the hospital and community health services (HCHS) budget by a weighted capitation formula. The English formula was origin-ally designed by the Resource Allocation Working Party in 1976 (Department of Health and Social Security, 1976), and this has recently been reviewed and refined by a team from the University of York (Carr-Hill *et al.*, 1994a, 1994b; Smith *et al.*, 1994). The refined formula uses the best available data and sophisticated statistical methods to identify population-based indicators of the need for health care using small area analysis of the determinants of hospital use.

This formula determines resource allocation between health authorities. However, the Department of Health decided to allocate only 76% of the total budget according to the new needs indices. This effectively prevented some redistribution of budgets away from the South and the Home Counties to the North of England. This decision created what was known as the 'mid-Surrey effect' owing to the coincidental benefit to the then Secretary of State's constituency! Box 2.7 illustrates the impact of this decision (Peacock and Smith, 1995). The validity of this partial application of the York formula is now accepted by bureaucrats and research-

Box 2.7
Winners and losers
from the partial
implementation of the
York formula

Bottom ten	Loss (%)	Top ten	Gain (%)
N.W. Durham	−3.55	Mid-Surrey	5.26
St Helens	−3.66	Wycombe	4.97
Salford	−3.70	S.W. Surrey	4.82
Barnsley	−3.71	W. Surrey	4.47
Durham	−3.74	N.W. Surrey	4.46
City & Hackney	−3.93	E. Surrey	4.34
Sunderland	−4.02	W. Berkshire	4.13
Liverpool	−4.20	Basingstoke	4.03
N. Manchester	−5.01	E. Hertfordshire	3.91
C. Manchester	−5.12	Tunbridge Wells	3.90

Source: Peacock, S. and Smith, P. (1995), *The Resource Alloca-tion Consequences of the New NHS Needs Formula*. University of York, Centre for Health Economics Discussion Paper 134: May.

ers as inappropriate (Brennan and Carr-Hill, 1996) and will, when politically opportune, be reversed.

The RAWP formula and subsequent refinements also apply only to hospital and community health services (HCHS) budgets, and not to primary care. The primary care budget is still largely demand determined and not cash limited: it is a function of the number of GPs and their prescribing behaviour. The individual GP's income is determined partially by a capitation formula (with some weight for age and social deprivation), but the efforts to equalize the distribution of GPs in different regions have been minimal, involving mostly 'negative directive' (the closing of 'overdoctored' areas to new entrants). Consequently, there are considerable inequalities in the distribution of primary care funding, and inequalities in access to primary care (the gatekeeper to the NHS). 'RAWPing' primary care budgets would have a significant impact on the distribution of budgets and GPs (Box 2.8), but there is difficulty in identifying an efficient need weighting. Even if this was formal and agreed, the policy of equating the budget allocation may require a radical change in the GP contract, potentially replacing the independent contractor status with a salaried service (Bloor and Maynard, 1995).

An equitable distribution of resources should precede the further development of managed care in the UK. It is important to recognize the use of the word 'further': the internal market already has many of the characteristics of a managed care system. However, there are problems here and in the USA with the further development of such mechanisms because of the failure to evaluate and the uncertainty inherent in much of the advocacy of such schemes. In particular:

Box 2.8
The effect of 'RAWPing' primary care in the UK, using a 'needs' based formula

Region	Actual expenditure (£m)	Target expenditure (£m)	Gain (% actual expenditure)
Northern	358.2	392.6	9.61
Yorkshire	418.0	430.3	2.94
Trent	524.3	546.7	4.27
E. Anglian	233.0	216.3	−7.17
N.W. Thames	393.9	359.5	−8.74
N.E. Thames	424.9	408.9	−3.76
S.E. Thames	408.3	400.1	−2.02
S.W. Thames	319.2	310.7	−2.66
Wessex	320.9	311.9	−2.81
Oxford	271.2	264.5	−2.46
S. Western	405.1	348.5	−13.97
W. Midlands	574.0	613.9	6.94
Mersey	286.2	294.3	2.81
N. Western	468.1	507.2	8.36

Source: Bloor, K. and Maynard, A. (1995), *Equity in Primary Care*. University of York, Centre for Health Economics Discussion Paper 141: October.

1. Will efforts to reduce utilization and cut variations in clinical practice reduce the quality of care? During the last decade, 'efficiency savings' in the NHS hospital sector has driven up activity levels with, generally, inpatient numbers being static and a rapid increase in day case activity. However, variations in activity between doctors remain large (Audit Commission, 1996) and the scope for vigorous intervention by Trust managers, GP contractors and DHA purchasers remains considerable.

2. Efforts to reduce practice variations together with pressure on clinicians to adopt good practice identified by the Cochrane Centre and the NHS Centre for Reviews and Dissemination may yield significant savings. However, in many areas of clinical practice, the evidence base is absent and practice guidelines have to be devised by experts and consensus. As the American physician Alvin Feinstein warned, 'the agreement of experts has been the traditional source of all the errors through medical history' (Feinstein, 1988). Not only may guidelines have little basis in terms of effectiveness, but their authors also tend to ignore their resource consequences (e.g. Grimshaw and Russell, 1993). The vigorous and extensive use of guidelines, if not based on evidence of cost effectiveness and revised regularly, may set bad practices in concrete and institutionalize inefficiency!

3. The scope for improved resource utilization in the USA and UK health care systems is considerable. However, the relative scope in the UK may be less than across the Atlantic. In both health care systems the costs of reducing inefficiency will be considerable: better, if not more, 'grey suits' will be needed, as will investments in information technology. There is a risk that, without careful management, the costs of improving practice may reduce the gains from enhancing efficiency. Such careful management will require development of proper practices of outcome measurement. At present GPs and all other NHS decision makers tend to be driven by cost savings and fail to measure, like their managed care counterparts in the USA, the effects of their practices on patient outcomes (length and quality of life, in terms of physical, psychological and social well-being). Public and private agencies will have to integrate established quality of life measures, e.g. SF-36 (Garratt *et al.*, 1993) and EuroQol (Brooks, 1996) into their practices.

4. The radical changes inherent in managed care organizations imply reform of the GP contract. Independent contractor status may survive for some time in middle-class and rural areas, but change may come in urban, disadvantaged areas. Contracts may develop with practices rather than individual GPs, and contracts may become more specific, clearly defined and renewable subject to performance. Thus capitation would remain for the practice, but GPs may be paid salaries, like other providers in primary care.

5. The reason for changing payment systems is usually to improve incentives. The scope for doctor–nurse and other forms of substitution is considerable according to advocates. They may be right, but so far the evidence is poor (Richardson and Maynard, 1995). If they are correct, the challenge is to induce providers to exploit the knowledge base and alter practice to obtain better patient outcomes and/or lower costs. In the USA, the engine of change has been profit. The for-profit managed care industry has developed its market by aggressive contracting and by undercutting the not-for-profit organizations. Health care billionaires have been created as the inefficiencies of the US health care industry have been converted into personal profits. This has created concern about quality and much self-examination by the medical profession, faced by confusion of their role as patients' advocate by concern for personal gain.

In the UK, part of the equivalent issue is whether GP fundholders should be permitted to keep part of their surpluses as profits. Would such an incentive drive beneficial change more rapidly? In the USA and the UK such devices would have to be regulated carefully to avoid adverse effects on patients' health status and inappropriate use of public funds.

CONCLUSION In the USA, managed care has revolutionized the finance and provision of health care for employees and is now being extended to Medicare and other federal and state programmes. In the commercial sector, employers welcome this as a mechanism which has slowed or even (in the short term) reversed health care expenditure inflation. The nature of health care provision has been and continues to be revolutionized with the development of mechanisms (such as primary care gatekeeping) familiar to the British.

Lessons can be learnt from the US experience. In particular change can be much more rapid than has occurred in the UK in the last 10 years. Such change can create major losers (providers) and gainers (management and owners!). The further commercialization of health care in the USA raises major issues about regulation and about the quality of care, which, as in the UK, is poorly evaluated. In the USA, mergers are leading to the creation of large and powerful buyers and provider (e.g. hospital) groups. As the eighteenth century political economist Adam Smith (1776) remarked:

> *People of the same trade seldom meet together, even for merriment and diversion, but the conversation ends in a conspiracy against the publick, or in some contrivance to raise prices.*

The paradox is that if market mechanisms are deployed in health care and all other markets, more regulatory activity in needed. In both the USA and the UK, the regulatory framework is poorly evaluated and weak.

Managed care can teach lessons to UK policy makers, provided these lessons are evidence based. The hype and advocacy of managed care enthusiasts should be contained by cheerful scepticism in the UK. Managed care is interesting but its advocates should bring evidence rather than rhetoric to the policy-making debate.

SUMMARY

- ◆ Health care reform should be evaluated in relation to cost containment, efficiency and equity objectives.
- ◆ US health policy has historically created cost inflation, with little attention to equity, while the UK has prioritized equity issues and cost containment.
- ◆ Managed care consists of a variety of strategies to integrate finance and delivery of health care, and control utilization of health services and costs to improve efficiency.
- ◆ Health care in the UK has, since the creation of the NHS, been 'managed'.
- ◆ The 1991 reforms made contracting and purchasing more explicit. GP and total fundholders operate similarly to a mini-health maintenance organization.

♦ Private health insurers in the UK are increasingly using preferred providers, and enforcing protocols to control cost and quality, and reduce practice variations.
♦ Before managed care initiatives are implemented in the UK, it is necessary to ensure an equitable distribution of health care resources.

FURTHER READING

♦ Rivo M.L., Mays, H.L., Katzoff, J. and Kindig, D.A. (1996), Managed care: implications for the physician workforce and education. *JAMA* **274**: 712–715.

This summarizes differences between the variety of organizational forms of managed care.

♦ Miller, R.H. and Luft, H.S. (1994), Managed care plan performances since 1980. *JAMA* **271**: 1512–1519.

This article reviews evaluations of the performance of managed care plans.

♦ Maynard, A. and Bloor, K. (1996), Introducing a market to the United Kingdom National Health Service. *New England Journal of Medicine* **344**: 604–608.

This summarizes the UK market reforms and critically appraises evaluations of their impact on the objectives of the UK health care system.

REFERENCES

American Medical Association's Council on Ethical and Judicial Affairs (1995), Ethical issues in managed care. *JAMA* **273**: 330–335.
Andersen, T.F. and Mooney, G. (eds) (1990), *The Challenges of Medical Practice Variations*. Macmillan, London.
Audit Commission (1996), *The Doctor's Tale II*. HMSO, London.
Bloor, K. and Maynard, A. (1995), *Equity in Primary Care*. University of York, Centre for Health Economics Discussion Paper 141: October.
Brennan M. and Carr-Hill, R. (1996), *No Need to Weight Community Health Programmes for Resource Allocation?* University of York, Centre for Health Economics Discussion Paper 146.
Brooks R., with the EuroQol Group (1996), EuroQol ref: the current state of play. *Health Policy* **37**: 53–72.
Carr-Hill, R., Hardman, G., Peacock, S., Sheldon, T. and Smith, P. (1994a), Allocating resources to health authorities: a small area analysis of inpatient utilisation I, background and methods. *British Medical Journal* **309**: 1046–1049.
Carr-Hill, R., Hardman, G., Peacock, S., Sheldon, T.A. and Smith, P. (1994b), *A Formula for Distributing NHS Revenues Based on Small Area Use of Hospital Beds*. University of York, Centre for Health Economics.
Congressional Budget Office (1994), *An Analysis of the Managed Competition Act*. Washington DC.
Dawe, V. (1996), Health insurers prepare for war. *Hospital Doctor* 23 May: 18.

Department of Health (1994), *Health and Personal Social Services Statistics for England*. HMSO, London.

Department of Health and Social Security (1989), *Working for Patients*. HMSO, London.

Department of Health and Social Security (1976), *Report of the Resource Allocation Working Party*. HMSO, London.

Enthoven, A. (1993), Why managed care has failed to contain health costs. *Health Affairs* Fall: 27–43.

Feinstein A. (1988), Fraud, distortion, delusion and consensus: the problems of human and natural deception in epidemiology studies. *American Journal of Medicine* **84**: 475–478.

Folland, S., Goodman, A.C. and Stano, M. (1993), *The Economics of Health and Health Care*. Macmillan, New York.

Friedman, E. (1996), Capitation, integration and managed care: lessons from early experiments. *JAMA* **275**: 957–962.

Fuchs, V. (1974), *Who Shall Live?* Basic Books, New York.

Garratt, A.M., Ruta, D.A., Abdalla, M.I., Buckingham, J.K. and Russell, I.T. (1993), The SF-36 health survey questionnaire: an outcome measure suitable for routine use within the NHS. *British Medical Journal* **306**: 1440–1444.

Gray, B.H. and Schlesinger, M. (1996), *The Profit Transformation of the Hospital and HMO Fields*. Paper presented for the Milbank Memorial Fund and Hospital Trustees of New York State: May 16.

Grimshaw, J.M. and Russell, I.T. (1993), Effect of clinical guidelines on medical practice. A systematic review of rigorous evaluations. *Lancet* **342**: 1317–1322.

Hiebert-White, J. (1995), Managed care and the new economics of mental health. *Health Affairs* **14**(3): 5–6.

Iglehart, J. (1994), Physicians and the growth of managed care. *New England Journal of Medicine* **331**: 1167–1171.

Kassirer, J. (1995), Managed care and the morality of the marketplace. *New England Journal of Medicine* **333**: 50–52.

Klein, R. (1993), Health care reform: the global search for Utopia. *British Medical Journal* **307**: 752.

Luft, H.S. (1981), *Health Maintenance Organisations: Dimensions of Performance*. John Wiley, New York.

Manning, W.G. *et al.* (1984), A controlled trial of the effect of a prepaid group practice on use of services. *New England Journal of Medicine* **310**: 1505–1510.

Marinker, M. (1984), Developments in primary health care. In Teeling Smith, G. (ed.) *A New NHS Act for 1996?* Office of Health Economics, London.

Maynard, A.K. (1986), Performance incentives in general practice. In Teeling Smith, G. (ed.) *Health Education and General Practice*. Office of Health Economics, London.

Maynard, A. and Bloor, K. (1995), Health care reform: informing difficult choices. *International Journal of Health Planning and Management* **10**: 247–264.

Maynard, A.K., Marinker, M. and Pereira Gray, D. (1986), The doctor, the patient and their contract III – alternative contracts are viable? *British Medical Journal* **292**: 1438–1440.

McPherson, K., Wennberg, J.E., Hovind, O.B. and Clifford, P. (1982), Small area variations in the use of common surgical procedures: an international comparison of New England, England, and Norway. *New England Journal of Medicine* **307**: 1310–1314.

Miller, R.H. and Luft, H.S. (1994), Managed care plan performance since 1980. *JAMA* **271**: 1512–1519.

NHS Executive (1996), A national framework for the provision of secondary care within general practice. *HSG*(96)31: 13 May.

Office of Health Economics (1995), *OHE Compendium 1995*. London, OHE.

Organisation for Economic Co-operation and Development (1994), *OECD Economic Surveys 1993–94*: United Kingdom. OECD, Paris.

Peacock, S. and Smith, P. (1995), *The Resource Allocation Consequences of the New NHS Needs Formula*. University of York, Centre for Health Economics Discussion Paper 134: May.

Richardson, G. and Maynard, A. (1995), Fewer doctors? More nurses? A review of the knowledge base of doctor–nurse substitution. Centre for Health Economics Discussion Paper 135. University of York.

Rivo, M.L., Mays, H.L., Katzoff, J. and Kindig, D.A. (1996), Managed care: implications for the physician workforce and education. *JAMA* **274**: 712–715.

Rogers, M.C., Synderman, R. and Rogers, E.L. (1994), Cultural and organisational implications of academic managed-care networks. *New England Journal of Medicine* **331**: 1374–1377.

Schroeder, S. (1996), The medically uninsured – will they always be with us? *New England Journal of Medicine* **334**: 1130–1133.

Smith, A. (1776), *Wealth of Nations*.

Smith, P., Sheldon, T.A., Carr-Hill, R., Hardman, G., Martin, S. and Peacock, S. (1994), Allocating resources to health authorities: a small area analysis of inpatient utilisation II: results and policy implications. *British Medical Journal* **309**: 1050–1054.

USA Today (1995), Some say HMOs come up short in specialized care. 17 October.

Weiner, J.P. (1994), Forecasting the effects of health reform on US physician workforce requirement. *JAMA* **272**: 222–230.

Wennberg, J.E., Freeman, J.L. and Culp, W.J. (1987), Are hospital services rationed in New Haven or over-utilised in Boston? *Lancet* **187**(8453): 1185–1189.

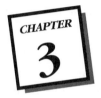

ETHICS OF PRIMARY HEALTH CARE

Roger Higgs

OBJECTIVES

♦ To explore the ethical dilemmas facing those involved in primary health care delivery.

♦ To understand the nature of an ethical dilemma, its origins and effects.

♦ To understand what is special about moral conflicts in primary care.

♦ To develop skills in moral management that can be used in practice.

INTRODUCTION Neither medicine nor management are purely technical areas to be solved just by the careful use of factual knowledge. Both require judgement and choice, and that implies examining values, looking at what is good or less good in a broader context, and negotiating between different outcomes or processes. This involves using moral reasoning as an integrated part of our practical skills.

In management we shall sometimes be presented with an obvious dilemma, well known and even clearly labelled, but the issues may be more hidden. Situations which make us feel morally uncertain or uncomfortable seem to be increasing. Certainly in primary care there are many occasions when we have to make apparently painful choices. So we need to be aware of the particular 'sensitive spots' in primary care and have good ways of identifying moral problems beforehand. We should have as clear a way of thinking about these as possible and be aware of our own prejudices. But, however clear our ideas are, they will always be challenged in practice, and there are some areas (such as confidentiality and teamwork, the best use of limited resources, advocacy and professional limits, and the management of medical advance and change), which require particular thought. It is likely that the last word will never be said about ethics in primary care. We need to be skilled and consciously trying to improve these skills as part of an integrated approach to patient-centred, holistic, team-based management.

ETHICAL
DILEMMAS

What is an ethical
dilemma?

In many years of working in this area, we have never come across anyone in primary care discussion groups who could not answer that question by providing an example. We all instinctively recognize issues that go beyond the purely technical, and pose problems for us in a wider context. You might wish to pause to think how you might answer. One way might be with a case: another might be something nearer a definition.

Clinical case 3.1
Setting the scene

> A young woman of 15 who wants to be a solicitor comes to see a male doctor just before her O levels. She comes from a family with little formal education, but is expected to do well. She presents with headaches, but it is clear that there is something really worrying her. She thinks she is pregnant and does not want to continue with the pregnancy. Her family are pillars of a local church which does not approve of abortion.
>
> While the nurse is testing the young woman's urine, the receptionist, in a slightly knowing voice which makes the doctor feel rather uncomfortable, tells him that her mother is on the phone and wants to speak to him urgently ...

The doctor knows that, since there was a recent 'pill scare' in the local press, there has been an unfortunate increase in requests for termination of pregnancy and there is now a long waiting list. The practice are not yet in control of the funds for abortion services.

Box 3.1
Clear issues

> A number of clear ethical issues arise from this case. We can all see the technical issues here: the diagnosis, how to get the patient on the waiting list as quickly as possible. We may also be aware of some legal problems, which might surround the future question of consent for an operation. But mostly what stands out for us are the ethical issues:
>
> ◆ How can we preserve patient confidentiality?
>
> ◆ How should I be consulting with someone who is in a legal sense under the age of consent?
>
> ◆ Is abortion right or wrong?

Ethical issues   There are both clear and unlabelled ethical issues raised by this case (Box 3.1).

These are questions which we probably recognize as falling within the orbit of medical ethics. We might know that there is already a body of writing about them. We could look them up.

However, there are also issues which are not so obvious (Box 3.2).

Box 3.2
Unlabelled issues

♦ Is termination of pregnancy something which should be part of the (free) national health service?

♦ If so, considering that it's an operation which is always better (in many senses) done sooner rather than later, is it fair that there should be a long waiting list?

♦ Is it right that people should receive information through the media which might mislead them or cause them harm?

♦ Whose choice is to be decisive or considered right if the patient, the parents and the doctor all disagree what to do?

These sort of questions are longer and perhaps slightly vaguer, but contains words such as 'right', 'better', and 'should'. These are neither truly medical nor clearly labelled ethical issues, but seem to be appealing to other ideas which lie behind them, such as equity, harm or respect for individual choice and self-rule. As we shall see, these are some of the principles, perspectives and values which mark out important ways of approaching moral discussion. Behind them yet further we might find the work of philosophers and thinkers in the field of ethics.

Moral discomfort   Fascinating as this last area might be, ordinary people have no need to delve deep into this academic field. We all have feelings which guide us towards what is right or warn use when something seems to be wrong. The doctor could tell that there was something more important on the young woman's mind than a nasty headache. The case as recounted indicates that the receptionist (her tone in speaking to the doctor being 'slightly knowing') had somehow picked up something of what is happening. The doctor's discomfort may arise from the problem of how to handle the call from the mother. It also may come from a feeling that perhaps the receptionist also being party to this confidential discussion is not somehow appropriate. Yet the nurse clearly knows what is going on; does the patient know that she knows? The doctor may even begin to feel cross that the mother is interfering, or upset and confused that there is something else going on that he does not understand; he may feel in some sense manipulated.

Thus a feeling of discomfort may lead us to detect problems which, up to that moment, did not have a 'moral' label, and may lead us to think twice about actions that previously would have been accepted without question. These feelings of something not being right, or other feeling like anger or disgust, are often the markers or reminders that there is a moral issue somewhere. Perhaps someone might claim that a sudden, unexpected and strong emotion coming up in clinical care or health care management is always the sign that there is a moral issue to be considered. What has usually happened is that something important has been allowed to go ahead without proper acknowledgement or discussion, or that some previous experience has not been resolved or sorted out. These are important concerns for everyone involved.

But they do not indicate clearly to us exactly what the problem is or how it should be resolved. This requires clear thinking.

Level of moral understanding and debate

So we can begin to see several ways in which ethical issues may enter health care. We begin to see a series of levels emerging (Box 3.3):

Box 3.3
Levels of moral understanding

Level 1	Moral discomfort	
1a	'Hey', 'No!' 'Whoops'	A feeling that something is not right or is unresolved
1b	Anger Disgust	A strong feeling as marker of a moral problem
1c	'That's not right but ... why not?'	A clear understanding of an (as yet un-named) moral problem
Level 2	**Moral dilemma**	
2	'A problem of confidentiality' 'I don't agree with abortion'	An ethical issue, explicit and identified
Level 3	**Moral principles**	
3	A framework of principles/ perspectives/values	
Level 4	**Moral philosophy**	
4	Philosophy/religion/ law, etc.	

In levels 2 and 3, we can see ways of beginning to handle the problems. No text books like this could do any more than point out the fourth level. It may be, however, that we can reach the third level in order to help us make sense of our decisions.

Moral health warning no. 1   One immediate warning is in order. You may have started reading this chapter hoping that you will be able to make sense of difficult decisions, and will be given guidance on how to go about that. We hope that too.

However, you will also notice that, in the process, other things which seemed resolved and sorted out may begin to be problematic. Just as it is the anthropologist's task to make the familiar strange, so ethical thinkers may find themselves making the accepted questionable. Things may get harder before they get easier. The only thing to do is to keep on reading and thinking.

Why should moral thinking be so important in management?   The example we used, of the pregnant teenager, may not be immediately obvious as a management issue. Yet some reflection will show how many management issues are contained within it, and the need for good moral thinking.

The doctor was a man. He may have been, and probably was, a sensitive, receptive individual and a good diagnostician. However, many young women in a similar situation might have preferred to see a woman GP; even to the extent of being put off coming to see the doctor. Would the availability of a woman doctor be a kindness, an important option or a right? How far should any organization, particularly based on small groups like primary care must be, make itself responsive to its users?

A person using a service may reasonably have some expectations of what he or she may receive from the service. If the service is itself not sure, the scene is set for some unpleasant confrontations between 'demanding' users and 'defensive' professionals. So the purposes of the service have to be clear. Clarification is not necessarily a moral task, but it is certainly often needed in thinking things through.

Purposes may derive from particular values which the service has or which the people who work in the service hold. These are often not explicit. The doctor, for instance, may feel that a young woman from this background who is a high flyer should have preferential treatment, or may see the need to preserve family integrity by being as open as possible. If these arguments are not open and available for discussion, patients and staff will be confused. We shall return to discussing values later.

Purposes and values may be clear, but no service can do everything for everybody. It has to have a clear set of priorities, and to have limits on its activities. This will require some policies to be made and some procedures to enable these policies to be put into effect.

The service may be clear about what it wants to do, and how, but this needs to be checked against the needs of those using the service. Here we return to our first question and come up against one of the biggest problems for any manager or provider of health care in the modern world. We can no longer assume, if we ever could, that we are dealing with people who share views about important things. In a modern multicultural and pluralistic environment, the unenviable task of a manager of health care is to provide for a whole range of needs, desires, purposes and expectations. This immediately begins to make explicit some of the virtues (in the sense of positive features or attitudes) that such a service should have. It has to think clearly about access, given people's different working and waking lives. It has to be tolerant of the different demands to be made on it. Although the individuals who work in it may need to be discriminating in the best sense, discrimination in its worse sense, that of prejudice like racism, agism or homophobia, should have no part in the structure.

Strangely, it is hard to find entries like 'racism' or 'homophobia' in medical ethics text books. The most optimistic explanation would be that racial tolerance, for instance, is basic to society at large, required by law in most Western countries, and so is not a specific issue for medical ethics. Yet we know that it is still a problem in health care, in the sense that some people experience it, and may, both as patients or professionals, worry that it may influence their judgement or the process of their care.

Moral health warning no. 2 Medical ethics is not some separate area of thinking on its own, with its own set of rules. It is part of moral thinking in general, that part of our lives where we all have to consider:

◆ Is this the best?
◆ Is this right?
◆ What should be done?

For the manager, these questions are not at the back but the front of the mind.

Are ethical issues a problem? For a clinician, running a good service as well must in some senses be more complex than just providing good personal care. Different skills are required. In that sense the manager also may need a differently tuned moral sensibility. However, there are other issues which suggest that being skilled in moral thinking may be increasingly important.

There is an increasing range of conditions for which the health service *could* offer a response but many of the new treatments are expensive, and every health service the world over is struggling with how best to use its limited resources. Political pressures are mounting everywhere for a debate or change in the way health services are run. However, professionals are becoming increasingly concerned about outside 'tinkering' by uninformed people in power with short term objectives, and financial constraints appear to be becoming more important than professional and clinical aims. People are better informed than ever before about what goes wrong with their minds or bodies, and what help they might expect from the health service. There is, however, no sign of much greater involvement of users in the planning or policy-making about health services, so there is evidence of increasing frustration and misunderstanding between patients and professionals.

As health care becomes more complex and responsive, different skills are required and teams are needed rather than just skilled individuals. But many of the standard ways of working depend on one-to-one relationships, and questions of professional power and limits of access to knowledge to preserve confidentiality become more complex. Luckily, most people seem to enjoy the process of becoming more ethically aware, and more skilled at detecting, thinking about and exploring moral issues. These issues identify some management conflicts (Box 3.4).

Box 3.4
Management conflicts

Individual vs team care
Political vs professional agendas
Financial vs clinical constraints
Holistic vs focused medical care
Patient satisfaction vs professional survival

MORAL CONFLICTS IN PRIMARY CARE   Many people would claim that changes in health services are the more obvious cause of conflict in primary care. This is usually voiced by the professionals. 'If only we were left alone to carry on as we used to, everything would be all right'. Sometimes, the same thought also comes from users. 'If only we could go back to the good old days, where we had the old family doctor who knew everything about us'. These statements often appear to ignore the changes that are happening elsewhere in society, to which the health service must respond, and to be guided by rosy memories rather than reality. However, they show real concerns about primary care of which every clinician and manager should take not. Change can easily become an end in itself or a routine management response to a problem. The cynic might say that change can be created as a cover for real progress: if things do not work out, a manager can either blame the process (rather than looking back to the original problem) or can be sure to be in another job by the time people realize that things have not improved. However, effective management must examine what were the characteristics of the service and how they answer clients' needs. In changing these, issues emerge which seem intrinsic to this part of the health service, and which may be revealed but not created by changes. We chose some of these as illustrations of typical and possibly intrinsic areas of moral choice about which a manager must be vigilant (Box 3.5).

Box 3.5
Areas of moral choice
in primary care

♦ *Communication:*
Diagnosis and treatment depend greatly on good com-munications, yet the factors which create good communi-cation (time, a good environment, reductions of tiredness and anxiety, professional training and reflection time) are expensive.

♦ *Access:*
It is difficult to control access for acute self-limiting condi-tions in primary care, yet good outcomes are largely the result of well-managed long-term conditions, which often excite less interest from professionals.

♦ *Patient relationship:*
Primary care professionals use their relationships with patients as one of their key forms of treatment, but this can be very tiring and induces stress.

♦ *Confidentiality:*
Staff often live near or amongst the patients they see, which makes confidentiality all the more important but even more difficult to achieve.

♦ *Uncertainty:*
Individuals vary in their ability to tolerate uncertainty, yet in primary care certainty is often difficult to achieve and roles have to be blurred.

IDENTIFYING MORAL PROBLEMS

In the current context of cost reduction and political or public pressure, and from the foregoing discussion, this may seem strange. There appears to be more than enough to be tackling without looking further. Faced with a difficult situation, clinicians and managers often understandably respond by looking at the technical side of a question. This is after all the area they were trained in and it is in some senses their expertise, but this ignores two vital aspects of management:

♦ We need to unpack the moral questions, and all the moral questions, in a particular issue, to see what should best be done.
♦ We need mechanisms for uncovering the other ethical concerns in the service.

Unpacking the Sometimes this work is taken further by *investigation*, sometimes
moral problems by *gathering data*, and sometimes by discussion and *thinking through* the questions.

Clinical case 3.1
Setting the scene
continues ...

> Having successfully fended off the mother, the doctor was perturbed by the waiting list of over a month to be seen for a termination of pregnancy for the schoolgirl. The reply to his telephone questions did not reassure him:
>
> > 'Well, to be frank doctor, we think the service is overwhelmed. I will pass your comments on to the management ... but I think priority has been given to the *real* and *deserving* aspects of our gynaecological service. After all, it's not as if contraception was not widely discussed and easily available nowadays is it? These young girls should take responsibility for what they do. Maybe she thought she could get a council place? Sorry, that's not fair is it? You want to speak to one of the consultants? Well, decisions are taken by management now. It's very hard to get anyone put up the list: that wouldn't be fair would it? And Mr Jenkinson isn't operating at the moment until he's better...'

The enquirer has been treated to a discussion going close to the heart of the service. What has been found has revealed a series of questions about the values of those running the service (Box 3.6). The reader may have others.

Box 3.6
Values and issues

> ◆ What are the responsibilities of those who run a service which is being 'overwhelmed'?
>
> ◆ How can one decide priority between different aspects of a health care system?
>
> ◆ Is there such a thing as a 'real and deserving' problem, or one that's clearly not?
>
> ◆ If the individual can prevent a problem, and does not or does so ineffectively, where does the financial responsibility for medical treatment lie?
>
> ◆ What should be done when a member of a public service reveals what appears to be unacceptable attitudes?

We shall shortly look at ways of structuring those questions. It is open to us also to check out some *facts*: perhaps in this case by looking at waiting times of our patients from secondary services (and of primary care patients for *that* service), or outcome of one service compared with another.

Uncovering other ethical concerns

Sometimes this work is taken further by: assessing the reaction of individuals; case discussion; carrying out audit and reviews; using patient participation groups; through external visits and complaints.

The *reaction of individuals* remains the beginning of most discussions of moral issues in management, but the manager's task will be at the least to enable such concern to surface and to be expressed. This depends to a degree on the style of management and culture of the organization. If professionals are restricted to 'obeying orders' in a top-down approach, or patients led to believe that compliance to professionals' instructions or time-scales is what matters most, it is unlikely that important ideas will come forward.

Clinical case 3.2
Setting the scene

> A student was sitting in with a nurse at a contraceptive session. 'This may seem a very naive question, but do you known who keeps that information and who has access to the computer records?' This started a discussion about record-keeping, registers and confidentiality in the primary care group which led to new guidelines and procedures.

This reminds us that the newcomer is always valuable, that good ideas may come from people not familiar with the system and that there needs to be a method of feeding concerns into the structure of an organization, however small.

Case discussion has always been a mainstay of professional education in primary care. Managers may need both to ensure that: there is dedicated time for this type of work; that the right (but not too narrow) spectrum of professionals is involved; and that the atmosphere enables participants to think broadly, to challenge established ideas and practices, and to reach the point where they can give a good account of why they think what they do think.

Clinical case 3.3
Setting the scene

> A group of doctors met with health visitor staff to discuss a disputed complaint of sexual abuse in a family in the practice. This case threatened to divide the professional team, as members 'took sides' between the different parties involved and, even in the discussion, individuals defended their own point of view until one of the women partners pointed out that she had begun to see things from the point of view of the child, and that those involved in the discussion had completely forgotten that it was the child's welfare that should be in the front of their minds.

This case reminds us that: imaginative thinking remains the key to good decision making; informal or formal role play can sometimes help a group make unexpected progress; and the moral searchlight should be turned on the person or group whose problems are *least* being considered.

Audit and routine reviews of various kinds are also part of any organization's checking mechanism.

Clinical case 3.4
Setting the scene

> A review of the work of a counsellor in a group practice was undertaken every 2 months with medical staff. No details were disclosed without permission of the patients, but overall patterns and problems were reviewed. At one meeting it was noted that the doctors were not referring anyone over the age of 55 to the counsellor. This revealed attitudes about personal change and development in the late middle aged and elderly that the professionals did not realize they held. It led to a change of referral style and referral procedure.

Lessons from this include: structured audits are vital for the health of an organization; but they should if possible allow for surprises and should lead to change; and they should be conducted or at least designed by those who have responsibility to make the system work.

Patient participation groups remain a popularly quoted way of including user views in an organization, and there is evidence that they are undervalued and underutilized. They can, however, occur in a range of formats, from the most formal to the loosest involvement for particular purposes.

Clinical case 3.5
Setting the scene

An advertisement in a group practice asked for a group of patients to declare themselves if they would be prepared to work with students in a teaching programme. An *ad hoc* group was established, which looked at how women's problems could be taught, and suggested new approaches to teaching and learning to be transmitted to the practice and the medical school. This led to input to the ethics programme as well as the clinical teaching.

Concerns of users should have high priority in any system and more is to be gained from involving users than professionals believe.

Complaints are unfortunately usually the way in which problems with ethical overtones come to light. Traditionally, professionals in health and social care feel extremely threatened by complaints and react in defensive mode. However, consumer groups have pointed out that, in other circumstances, enlightened corporations pay great attention to complaints as these are the way by which the system can be tested or 'proved', and by which defects in a product or in delivery can be brought to light and eliminated. Perhaps it is the 'investment of self' by the professional in health care which makes complaints problematic.

Clinical case 3.6
Setting the scene

A doctor and nurse team become steadily more embroiled with a 'problem' family which finally made a complaint about their care. The professionals initially reacted by threatening to strike the family off the list until the health service body suggested the use of a conciliator. With this new person's help, they were able to stop sending letters and to meet to discuss the problem. The family had had a previous poor experience of health care from a quite unrelated set of doctors which had made them very nervous of medical intervention and trustworthiness. This was not known to the new team, who could only see the family's attitude as one of 'ungracious ingratitude and worse' until the previous circumstances were revealed.

It is likely that a third party, with no investment in a complaint, is a necessity for achieving the right balance in a complaints procedure, and this should probably be done as close to the primary care team's work as possible. At the very least people with a grievance should be allowed their say. It is likely, in spite of the attitude of some insurance companies, that saying 'sorry' if there has been a mistake, explaining what went wrong and how the team intends to prevent it happening again are key to the practical issues of preventing complaints becoming more serious, and to the moral question of respecting individual's rights and autonomous requests.

Visits from external units are not part of most current British primary health care procedure, and many are glad of that. However, it is not clear to the outside world exactly how primary care is accountable to the public for its work and it seems likely that the service should give thought to this before others do it for them.

Clinical case 3.7
Setting the scene

> A visiting academic was asked to review the primary care service provided under contract in a foreign country. As expatriate doctors were used, translators were a necessity. The visitor asked to sit in on some consultations with permission. The first consultation seen was a young man, flanked by two friends, who was clearly very disturbed. He began to talk at length without the interpreter offering any translation. When the doctor protested, the interpreter said 'It is nothing important, it is just psychiatric'. The visitor noted on top of the list the recommendation that interpreters should have a formal course in the aims and methods of primary care.

FINDING A FRAMEWORK TO EXPLORE THE ISSUES

We have spent time considering the substance of moral concerns in management and how we pick up and identify the issues. We follow the thesis that this is in a real sense half the battle. Moral problems unidentified or denied have a way of lurking inside an organization, however small, which suggests analogies with individual or group psychotherapy. One family therapist has suggested that a denied emotion can go about like a disaffected band of troops in a campaign who suddenly seize on a piece of territory and create mayhem. Whether one likes the analogy or not, *systems theory* suggests that a particular dysfunction can present itself at all sorts of levels in an organization or structure, and it is likely that a moral issue may occur recurrently at different points in a similar way.

Clinical case 3.8
Setting the scene

A young woman who had a history of emotional abuse and chaotic parenting as a child began to find difficulties with her new young family when she had children. She presented with recurrent overdoses at the local accident and emergency department. The psychiatrist in charge after assessment decided she had no formal psychiatric illness. Following an admission when she appeared to threaten him he barred her from the hospital. She began to make chaos in primary care, turning up to the GP without appointments several times a week, repeatedly telephoning, declaring a threat to commit suicide to many different members of the primary care team. The practice organization was disrupted, she created difficulties in the partnership and indirectly caused a complaint to the FHSA and the local MP. Finally, she was brought into a regular relationship with two members of staff and the chaotic behaviour began to diminish.

This case reminds us that the framework of practice offered in conventional primary care may be as good as we are likely to get, but is neither the best or necessarily the last word in organization. Many people's real needs will not fit well into this particular system. Just as there will be limits to the usefulness of any organization for a particular individual, so there may be limits to any framework of thinking applied to the ethical issues in a management dilemma. We present an approach which will enable some progress to be made, however. This framework approaches the problems through three main dimensions (Box 3.7).

Box 3.7
Framework dimensions

◆ Major principles and their scope

◆ Values

◆ Perspectives, roles and responsibilities

Major principles and their scope   The approach currently enjoying most favour is medical ethics uses *major principles* as a method of analysis, and reviews the strength or balance of these in particular contexts. These principles are seen as underlying other concerns in health care. Although they have philosophical backing, they have also practical 'street credibility' and have been used widely in anglophile countries to provide bearing in ethical debate (Box 3.8).

Box 3.8
Major principles

- ◆ Respect for autonomy
- ◆ Beneficence (maximizing good)
- ◆ Non-maleficence (minimizing harm)
- ◆ Justice (fairness)

The other concerns we have noted so far can be illuminated with reference to these principles.

1. Respect for autonomy

This is often taken as the starting place in Western medicine as it enshrines a key approach, backed in most countries by the law. Baldly stated, this is that, whatever professionals may suggest, people have the right to have their own choices respected in health care in as far as these choices are about themselves as individuals. (This contrasts with the 'doctor knows best' approach of previous decades, which is a form of *paternalism* which suggests that the first and final word rests with the professional, not the patient.) The acceptance of the new concept is based on several key features of illness and health care.

A person usually (unless causing harm to others) has the choice as to whether to be a 'patient' in the first place. Once becoming so, both the technical approaches to medicine and the difficulties (physical and psychological) of making key medical judgements about oneself put at risk a patient's ability to actualize key decisions, hence the need to *respect* that *autonomy* (literally, self-rule). This does not extend to issues that do not directly concern the patient, but it determines that it is the patient's wishes which are normally to be respected unless that person is not *competent* to make the choice (viz. unconscious, mentally deranged, too young). A professional acting against a competent person's request or wishes might thus risk the legal charge of assault. From this key principle are derived the concerns of that individual expressed in other areas, like consent to treatment, confidentiality and definitions of need. The competency question, however, may be problematical: how young is too young, how mad is too mad, to have one's wishes respected? – and so on. Although the danger is there that one set of wishes may simply be substituted for another, the word 'respect' underlines that, whenever possible, other things being equal, such choice as a person is clearly *able* to make *is* respected, and that full recovery is linked with the return to competent decision-making capacity.

This principle, we should note, does not adjudicate between different claims: the young woman, the mother and the doctor in Clinical case 3.1 may all have claims to have their autonomous wishes respected. It would be the current law in UK that, although a 15 year old is below one of the legal ages for consent (there being different ages for different social functions), nevertheless, if a child knows what she is consenting to and understands it, she should be considered competent. A three year old, however, might be different, and a fetus might have difficulty in seeing its rights or claims protected. Although the doctor and mother have their own autonomy to be considered – each might reasonably refuse to be involved with a procedure she thought wrong, that would not normally overrule the decision made by another competent person about that other person's health.

2. Beneficence (doing good)

Problems may arise in health care particularly when one person can see that an individual's decisions about themselves may not be helping them as it should. In order to maximize benefit in general, there has been increasing discussion of *guidelines* (agreed beforehand about a group of patients or a particular condition), of *evidence-based medicine* (the best treatment as defined by research) and of *managed care*, where a system is set up with the best intentions of a group in mind. However, such generalizations – that people are best served if they stop smoking, that a bleeding person should have a transfusion, or that a diabetic should be maintained at such and such a weight – may well conflict with the autonomous choices of adult smoker, Jehovah's witness or overweight gourmet. This principle is vital in that it prevents professionals from choosing, let us say, to give a cheap treatment which is ineffective, or to go off duty at a vital moment when there is no one to relieve them in the case of severe critical illness. It does, however, depend on a clear agreement from that person that he or she is indeed a patient, and agrees to be so.

There is no doubt that we all make priorities in our thinking. The administrator who rated 'real gynaecological work' higher than termination of pregnancy, or the doctor who considers the case of a bright child from a deprived background as more worthy of NHS care than someone who had a less productive future, are extreme and perhaps in some eyes examples of poor ethical thinking. However, they make the point.

One of the problems here may be the clash between *general* and *individual welfare*. Welfare programmes, however well researched or designed and however closely related to 'real' need, have to make broad decisions about what is best for people. The question remains about an individual's ability to opt out, but a second question goes to the heart of philosophy. Some people consider what it 'best' to be that which gives in some senses the greatest good to the greatest number (utilitarianism) or to depend on the *outcomes* or *consequences*. This type of thinking, which looks forward, can be contrasted with decisions based on *duties* or *rights* (deontological thinking) which is seen in some senses to look back. These approaches may agree. An example might be informed consent, where studies show that patients who know what to expect usually have a better outcome, but often they are in tension or opposition, such as in medical research. Here, the greatest good for the greatest number might well be to do limited but clear experiments on a group of people, whatever their views, in order to benefit others, but this is kept in check by concerns about autonomy. (A thoughtful utilitarian might still respond by pointing out that choice in this context preserves trust and thus overall creates a better world.) Most of us use a mixture of these two approaches, looking at outcome or duties as appropriate in different circumstances, but we should be aware of the different results that might follow if we were to change the style or structure of the argument.

3. Non-maleficience or minimizing harm

One of the main motives for a professional to intervene against a person's wishes is in order to avoid or prevent a clear harm. Thus a schizophrenic, intent on killing someone who is falsely seen by the patient as being a polluting evil in society, should be restrained. Parents who are injuring a child under their care are to be prevented from doing so. An epileptic who has daytime fits should be prevented from driving. This is now, conversely, seen as a responsibility on the professional to act in order to prevent harm. The same would apply to a manager: someone who allowed a dangerous employee to stay at work or a harmful system to continue to function without taking remedial action would be considered to be at fault. Key questions might be, how dangerous, how harmful, and who would judge that? Each of us might have different views of what constitutes a harm, and how different harms or risks might be graded in a particular case (such as in the case of removing a child from his or her home or stopping an HIV-positive employee from working in an operating theatre).

4. Justice or fairness

It could be said that autonomy, beneficence, and non-maleficence are good moral ends in themselves whereas justice seems more like a means to an end. In the narrow sense of *retributive* justice is may be, but in the other form, *distributive* justice, we do more than just encompass outcomes. We shall be largely concerned with the latter, although we may assume that no good manager would wish to take a quietistic attitude to criminal, antisocial or immoral behaviour. Our main concern, in management, as the millennium turns, is how to achieve a proper distribution of the resources available for health care. If once these were seen as limitless, they are now clearly considered finite by most societies: there is a limit to what people are prepared to contribute from their pockets for public and individual health, even their own.

A step back will allow us to recognize that the process of illness, disease or accident may be seen as inherently unjust. We might say of someone who overworks or smokes like a chimney that 'they deserve to get ill', but in that we can also see others doing the same who do not get ill life seems unfair. What is applicable to illness is even more so when it comes to inherited or genetic disorder and accidents. That Jack suffers and Jill does not, or vice versa, is one reason why some do not believe in a benign deity, and is the very reason why we need morality in the first place. As G.J. Warnock remarked 'There is in what may be called the human predicament a certain "natural" tendency for things to go very badly'.

Suffering deserves a response, but for many reasons it often does not get it. Yet selfless behaviour is needed by society for its survival and one of its modes of operation, in its broadest sense, is morality. Because we do not all start from the same line, in terms of genetic endowment and circumstances of birth as well as future lifestyle, we need a health *service*. Such a service aims to allow everyone to reach his or her *full potential*, not just repair the ills that befall people on the way. Such a service was envisaged in the British NHS and in the statements of the World Health Organization. These aims are broad and perhaps impossibly idealistic, but even before we discuss specific priorities, we have to notice general conflicts, such as between the demands for effort and expenditure on *prevention* as against *cure*, or on *acute* as against *long-term* conditions, *accidents* versus *disability*, or *physical* balanced against *mental* disorders.

Are resources finite, and in what sense? One of the ways in which the debate has recently been narrowed is by suggesting that resources are largely, as economic entities, what we can afford, about wealth or poverty, and who will pay. Other resources available to us hardly receive a mention. However, there are *human resources*, in terms of people to help in curing or caring. Yet again the debate emphasizes the cost and thus the rarity of trained professionals, and fails to see that there are huge human resources available in families and self-care, which remain untapped or underdeveloped. Some have seen the development of professional care as itself a sickening process because ordinary people become disempowered and lose the confidence to look after themselves. Equally, the positive human resources even in professionals of, for example, *commitment* and *enthusiasm* have been poorly discussed.

Given all this, however, we can assume that we are now all alerted to the restricted resources available for health care, and the consequent need to consider rationing in some form or other. How can this be done?

Scope or limits

It is time to consider both the *scope* or *limits* of these principles first. Simply stated, we can say that these principles only extend to those entities and those circumstances which are relevant to health care, that is, in the first place to people, and in the second to issues concerning health and disease. We probably understand what a person is or is not: we know a tree or house is not a person, although we might begin to waver about our own dog or cat. Much more difficult is the question of a fetus or early embryo, or a dead body. What claims on us do they have, to respect, avoid harming, and so on? Detail must be all important here, but also is a matter for personal judgement and disagreement. Yet law and policy must decide, and management with them. Who has access to a dead person's medical records and for what purpose? What should our response be to people with strong views, either way, about abortion or euthanasia?

Returning to resources, the second issue is the key: what are the limits to *care* and, specifically, what are the limits to *health* care? Is infertility a health care issue, sometimes, always or never to be funded from the public or the private purse? The same question can be asked of counselling or cosmetic surgery? Some progress at least can be made by being clearer about what we mean by a threat to health.

It might be important to visit important areas to clarify the debate. Underpinning the approach of primary care is what might be called the principle of *parsimony*: that is, that one should, between equally effective investigations or treatments, other things being equal, choose the cheapest one to use, and that new procedures should have to prove that they have something else to offer as benefit over current practice if they have a higher cost.

However obvious this may be, primary care has an honourable record, and one to maintain, in this area. If something can be diagnosed cheaply with a major and appropriate degree of accuracy, then further expenditure is inappropriate and wasteful. We abandon the clinical confidence we associate with, say, the diagnosis of an anxiety headache or a heart attack in primary care at the peril of unnecessary cost.

We return to the conflict between public health and individual care. What might be seen as 'best thing' for a group might not suit the preference of an individual. It is for this reason that public health is a separate function in the current health service, and one of the reasons why British GP fund holding, where the same person may make judgements both about what *groups* of people or conditions should be funded and which *individuals* should be put forward for care, has seemed to some people problematic. The American law academic Rawls was trying to make a similar point about distributive justice when he suggested that ideally the decisions about who should receive what should be made behind a 'veil of ignorance'. This meant that the people who were making such decisions were not able to know or predict what their own needs in the system might be. Although the situation is slightly different, the question of *detachment* remains important. The distinction between the public health decisions (about the group, or the service overall) and personal decisions (individual, tailored, advocated) appears to be healthy and important. Just as we do not like the judge and jury to be combined, nor perhaps should the public health and personal advocacy. If our commissioning processes threaten them, we should, in primary care, try to divide them again.

In situations where groups in society have to make difficult choices, Western countries have developed some form of process of debate amongst people, or amongst representatives of people, albeit with different rules and variable success. When it comes to individual decisions, rules in health care have become quite stringent about consulting the individual who matters most – the patient – and respecting her or his autonomous decision. With decisions about groups, some form of public control or accountability is traced back to health authorities and their public health departments. If a locality decides varicose vein surgery is not on the list, it is possible to disagree, lobby, campaign and so on. It is not clear, however, what links exist between the public and public health or resource decisions taken in general practice or primary care.

The well-known experiment in taking resourcing decisions to the people was that of the state of Oregon in the USA. In a large campaign of meetings, phone calls, focus groups and debates, people were asked to rank health care interventions, and a formula was used to create a prioritized list. This could be costed and a line drawn at that point where public finance would no longer be available because of total cost. The campaign has been criticized on technical grounds, and because it had unrealistic expectations of lay judgements about the effectiveness of different health care manoeuvres. But at least it was explicit and the public were involved.

A number of different instruments have been devised, most by health economists, to compare outcomes of different procedures in order to try to find the best value for money. Perhaps the best known entity in this field is the QALY, or 'quality adjusted life-year'. Here a year of healthy life expectancy is worth 1, and less healthy lives will have scores of less than 1 (being dead is worth 0). Although this may seem crude, it does give a quantification which can then be attached to each type of intervention, and, the argument runs, different interventions can then be compared. The problems of this type of approach are many: they cannot compare individual cases, and they do seem to ignore many of the values which would normally be brought into play including our complex but important understanding of 'need'. Judgemental comparisons, uncomfortable though they may be, still have to be made.

Values   The risk implicit in health economics, however carefully and cleverly performed, is that we shall known the cost of everything but still not the value of anything. Actuarial statistics can tell us the financial figure associated with the loss of a human life of a particular age and so on, but not the value to each of us if the life was that of someone we loved dearly. That person is scarcely replaceable, even if the role (breadwinner, carer) may be able to be costed. In the same way we all have values, derived from our society or culture, our family, our education, our life plans, which individually belong to us.

Clinical case 3.9

> A retired cricketer lost his wife when he was 72. At 78 he developed intermittent claudication, and rest pain a year later, closely followed by incipient gangrene of one leg. The surgeon strongly advised amputation; the patient declared he would rather die. The surgeon introduced him to successful amputees, and declared that he thought he was depressed because he was toxic, and therefore not competent to make the decision. The patient was adamant that as a sportsman his legs were vital to him. Legal action was threatened on both sides, and the leg began to rot. Conciliation was achieved through the GP obtaining a visit from a geriatrician, who suggested the man was dying, not just the leg. Good terminal care allowed the old sportsman a few days of peace before he died.

Just as individuals may have clear (but usually not explicit until challenged) hierarchies of values, so may institutions. These are likely to have a different pattern from those of the workers in the institution, even from the professional leaders. Conflict may occur between the value set of the institution, such as a GP practice, and those who work in it.

Perspectives,   People may 'play different parts' in their lives as they get older, but
roles and   they may also have different roles at the same moment of their lives.
responsibilities   They must adjust properties according to the particular role being undertaken and the responsibility given to that role. The perspective of patient, carer, relative at a distance, district nurse or doctor may all be different:

Clinical case 3.10

An elderly women with a lifetime label of schizophrenia was looked after by the local publican whose inn was next door to her house. There were rumours of a long-term attachment. The other (and recent) tenant in the house become increasingly disturbed as the old lady's hygiene deteriorated and she began to leave gas and water taps on. Her nearest relative, a daughter living 30 miles away with a handicapped child, seemed unnaturally eager to get the old lady into long-term institutional care and realize the asset of the house in a now 'gentrified' part of London. The district nurse saw a deterioration in the patient's self-care and felt he was being asked to undertake too many visits for too little benefit, and urged the GP to get her into hospital. The GP could not per-suade the old lady to move, and felt there was nothing, bar her previous diagnosis, which would allow her removal under public health or mental health legislation. The GP also was very touched by the publican's devotion. One Christmas, the tenant was away, the publican was ill and the old lady's flat was burgled. She died of hypo-thermia. Relations between doctor and district nurse also became very cold.

Equally, one individual may carry different roles, which may cause conflict. We are used to considering, though perhaps not resolving, the conflicts between a professional role and that of parent or home partner. However, at work, a primary care profes-sional may be clinician, teacher, friend, employer, manager, busi-ness partner, health service planner, researcher and so on. These individual roles may be in conflict.

Clinical case 3.11

A long-term and much liked receptionist began to arrive late for work and made some unusual decisions. No one was sure what was happening. Sensitive questioning was blocked. The petty cash began not to add up. One day a couple with an adopted child complained that she had stopped them and made peculiar accusations to them about things she could not have known without looking into the medical records. The partnership were divided about whether she should be sacked, until they received a formal complaint via the FHSA from the couple.

CONCLUSION The manager must be able to see the moral components in problems which present. Whether these need to be addressed or not, to fail to notice them at all will lay up trouble ahead. Because management is often about conflict, we should expect moral conflict too, especially in primary care, which has to take on board the aims and aspirations of so many different and disparate people and systems of work or thought. Ethical insights often work by posing questions, and only if the question is right can we be sure of getting near to the best answer. Some questions are given in Box 3.9 (p. 67). A moral dilemma may contain many different aspects. Our suggestion is that a 'cut' using the three different dimensions discussed, exercising the balance or conflict between the major principles and the limits or scope of their use, the values of the group (related to its task) and the individuals who are concerned, and the perspectives, roles and responsibilities of the various players or stakeholders, will enable a rounded assessment to be formed.

Box 3.9
Some questions for managers

♦ Is this situation just requiring a technical approach, or is there a broader moral question contained within it?

♦ Can I be clearer about what those moral questions or issues might be?

♦ Is anything or anyone trying to obscure those moral issues, and if so why?

♦ Whose voice is currently least heard in this debate and why? How can we hear what this voice wants to say?

♦ What principles operate here, and what are their limits?

♦ What are the key values of the institution and the individuals in this situation?

♦ What are my own emotional reactions and my personal value set?

♦ What role am I currently in and who am I working for?

♦ What resources are in scarce supply and can they be obtained in another way?

♦ Should the decision-making process be set up in a different way? Are the voices of individuals, professionals and the public each receiving attention?

♦ Is there a technical or economic assessment which is relevant?

SUMMARY

In order to manage well and achieve good results a manager should:

♦ Be alert to the moral issues raised by any problem.
♦ Know how to identify and describe the moral aspects of a problem and the possible effects of failing to do so.
♦ Have a language and framework with which these issues can be handled and put them to use.
♦ Be explicit with self and others about all the above.
♦ Develop skills as a lifetime process in the identification, assessment and management of medico-moral issues in health care.

FURTHER READING

♦ Gillon, R. (1994), *Principles of Health Care Ethics*. Wiley, Chichester.

This is the 'big book' which brings together many of the good contributors in medical ethics for the UK market. Its title shows its bias, but it is well referenced and does not duck debate. It is not one to read at one (or even several) sittings, so the following smaller books are also suggested.

♦ Campbell, A. and Higgs, R. (1982), *In That Case*. Darton Longman and Todd, London.

This is brief and readable, and looks at actual problems through different perspectives, following one case history through and deriving the theories from it. It is more about how to do it, and less about theory.

♦ Pratt, J. (1995), *Practitioners and Practices: a conflict of values?* Radcliffe Medical Press, Oxford.

This looks at the many conflicts raised by new styles of medicine and management in primary care. Clear and team-based.

♦ Toon, P. (1994), *What is Good General Practice?* Royal College of General Practitioners, London.

This is one of the RCGP Occasional Papers, and is a stimulating response to the question in the title.

♦ Boyd, K., Higgs, R. and Pinching, A. (1997), *The New Dictionary of Medical Ethics*. British Medical Journal, London.

This brings together the huge range of issues and responses now available, in a format which allows brief reading and expanding connections to take the reader on.

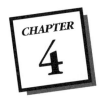

PRACTICE OBJECTIVES, PLANNING AND STRATEGY

Carolyn Semple Piggot

Carolyn Semple Piggot

OBJECTIVES

- ◆ To explore the nature of planning and its relevance to particular activities within general practice.

- ◆ To examine past performance and current decision making, in evaluating future needs.

- ◆ To define and explain strategic and operational planning, and tools by which planning processes may be achieved.

- ◆ To identify practice needs and requirements to facilitate this process.

- ◆ To identify quality and performance indicators by which results and progress can be measured.

INTRODUCTION

Planning is recognizably part of current general practice. It is important for the work and development of the practice. For example, general practice fundholders are required to submit plans for proposed expenditure and services each year, in addition to the annual report. With over 50% of the population in the UK covered by the fundholding scheme, interest in the planning process has increased. Plans go beyond bids for General Medical Services (GMS) monies (improvements to premises or bids for additional staff) to record the detailed planned use of National Health Service (NHS) and practice assets.

Fundamentally, planning entails managing change. This, of course, is familiar; if only in a domestic context (such as moving house, buying a new car or going on holiday). When it comes to thinking of planning in the practice context, it may be less so. Having a structure for the planning process acts as a prompt for the steps which make the production of the plan easier. As with planning for a family holiday, all members of the 'team' should be involved, bringing a useful range of views to the discussion.

This chapter looks at planning (called in some parts of the country, practice development planning), at tools and techniques to help in the planning process, and distinguishes between strategic and operational planning.

Operational plans   Operational plans are often easier; looking at the short term, with an emphasis on actions. Their focus is usually internal – what is going on inside the organization or practice. An example of this type of plan is the introduction of a new appointment system, a crucial part of an efficiently run practice. Another example is the retirement of a partner. Ideally, this would require several years' planning to ensure a smooth changeover. This plan could consider the development and training of staff and partners. This will enable the practice to meet the challenges of the future more easily and support the changes needed for the integration of a new staff member into the practice.

Strategic plans   Strategic planning has an external focus in which the changes in the environment are considered in terms of the impact they will have on the practice. It is this area which is commonly less well developed in the health service. An example of this is the development of commissioning in partnership with the health authority or health board, or with other practices. This will involve the practice in additional workload and needs to be integrated with other practice activities.

The first part of the chapter looks at what planning is and why it is useful, to provide a context for the planning process. Next, the chapter looks at the planning process itself, a core part of the planning framework, with examples taken from practice plans across the country. This will include checklists. The framework includes environmental analysis, SWOT, key issues, critical success factors, objectives, action plans and monitoring performance, as shown in Figure 4.1. It also looks at contingency planning and risk management. Visions and mission statements will be addressed, as applied to the NHS and, particularly to general practice. This part will also include a discussion of the values which drive decision making. The planning process includes a consideration of the resources to be used (people, money and time), so these will be covered, including how they can be integrated into the plan.

The chapter will then cover the issue of quality and performance measurement – as milestones and outputs are important in determining how well the practice is doing against the plan. The participation of the practice team will be an important part of the planning process, and contribute to the success or failure of the plan. The chapter will finish with a summary of key points.

Figure 4.1
An integrated planning
process

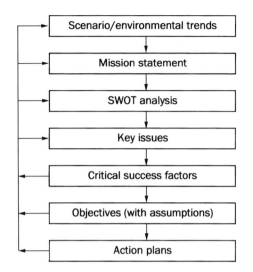

Scenario/environmental trends

Mission statement

SWOT analysis

Key issues

Critical success factors

Objectives (with assumptions)

Action plans

Source: Semple Piggot, C.
(1996), *Business Planning
for NHS Managers.* Kogan
Page, London, reproduced
with permission.

**WHAT IS
PLANNING?**

*An aircraft pilot would be barred and criminally prosecuted if he
took off without a flight plan.* (Dixon, personal communication)

Taking a car journey to a strange town or city involves first
consulting a map which would provide information on which to
plan the route. Despite this, many business and life decisions are
taken with far less planning and preparation. Every organization,
including general practice, needs a 'route map' which will help it to
see its destination, work out the best way to get there and, more
importantly, to identify when it has arrived.

Key elements   Planning involves the following key elements:

◆ Deciding where the organization currently is.
◆ Deciding what it is that needs to be achieved.
◆ Thinking ahead.
◆ Looking at the wider picture.
◆ Monitoring the progress of the practice.
◆ Planning for, rather than reacting to, events.

To help in organizing ideas for the plan, there are four key
planning questions (Box 4.1).

Box 4.1
Key questions in
planning

◆ Where are we now?

◆ Where do we want to be?

◆ How can we get there?

◆ How will we know when we have arrived?

Figure 4.2
The health gain cycle

Source: Roe, P. and
Semple Piggot, C. (1994),
*Health Gain and How to
Achieve it*, reproduced
with permission from
Glaxo Wellcome, UK.

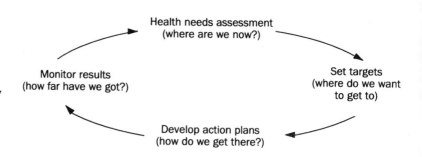

Health needs assessment
(where are we now?)

Set targets
(where do we want
to get to)

Monitor results
(how far have we got?)

Develop action plans
(how do we get there?)

Before putting pen to paper, these questions need to be thought about, together with the resources available to make the plan happen. In a health service context, these planning questions can have a more specific meaning. It may be helpful for the practice to consider the planning questions in terms of the health gain cycle (Figure 4.2), as it will focus the team on the services required to meet the needs of patients.

Purpose of plans   Planning should not be regarded as a one-off exercise. Neither should it be seen as simply producing a business plan for presentation to the health authority or health board as a way of bidding for resources. Planning should become part of the practice's culture, fundamental to the way in which the practice copes with the changes happening in the health care environment.

Planning is a continuing process. It involves looking both at what is going on within the practice and also to its environment. The process can identify the best opportunities for practice development, where innovations to services can be made for the benefit of patients and where the risks to the practice may be, together with ideas for how these can be tackled. Planning, therefore, considers both the health gain for patients and a more secure future for the practice.

WHY PLAN?   The challenges for general practice are great. Since the inception of

The need for   the NHS, there has been a move from single-handed practices to

planning in the   group practices, employing several ancillary staff. One of the key

1990s   current environmental catalysts for change in the 1990s is the move towards a 'primary care-led NHS'. The definition of what this actually means may vary, depending on who is doing the planning, but the aim is to provide general practitioners (GPs) with the ability to exert a much greater influence on the pattern of health services locally, to move resources from the traditionally powerful secondary care sector to primary- and community-based settings and to make the most of the trend towards evidence-based decision-making, particularly in the field of clinical care and the practice of medicine. Of course, this latter initiative includes the application of individual clinical judgement to individual patient cases – it is rare that a patient will present to the doctor as a text-book case to be dealt with in rigid adherence to an inflexible protocol. A further factor in the NHS environment is the need for a close working relationship between health and social services. GPs are asked to become increasingly concerned with the wider aspects of patient care, which requires close cooperation between a number of agencies.

So a plan is essential to ensure that resources are deployed to the best advantage for effective and efficient patient care, with health care applied appropriately on an equitable basis, ensuring access for those patients who need it and meeting the criteria for social acceptability. The plan offers a framework for this decision-making process.

Value of plans   A number of people have a vested interest in the success of the practice – its staff, its patients, the health authority or health board, and the suppliers of its specialized services. The plan is, therefore, a tool to communicate the future intentions of the practice. This will enable these people to understand and support the direction in which the practice is moving. It will also provide a basis for bidding for and using resources to best effect, identify specific roles and responsibilities for members of the practice. It will also consider the timescales over which the changes will take place, and identify the performance standards against which the practice's progress towards its objectives can be measured.

FORMAT OF A   Before the plan is written, it is worth checking that the elements of
'GOOD' PLAN   an effective plan are included. The length of the planning document should indicate that it is substantial enough to provide a clear indication of the intentions of the practice, without being overlong. Conciseness is appreciated by the reader. All well-prepared plans have a purpose.

For example, one practice has defined its mission statement as 'Our aim is to provide a friendly and efficient service to our patients, giving them easy access to high-quality and sensitive care'.

A plan should show that the purpose can be achieved. It is, therefore, important to explain how the objectives will be met, by describing action plans. Recommendations for action should be clearly defined and the reason for the choice explained for the reader. The plan should identify the results expected from the chosen course of action. That way, surprises are minimized. If the plan includes specific actions for practice staff, those responsibilities should be allocated. It provides a useful starting point for job descriptions and individual objectives.

A summary of the outcome of the planning process is shown in Box 4.2.

Box 4.2
The planning process
outcome

- ◆ A statement of aims and objectives.
- ◆ Crystallization of thoughts.
- ◆ Teambuilding.
- ◆ Motivation of the practice team which also strengthens the team spirit.
- ◆ A planning tool for the future.
- ◆ A statement of practice finance.
- ◆ Resource planning and bidding.
- ◆ Audit procedures to check progress.
- ◆ The chance to discuss and plan for the management of change.
- ◆ A way to achieve practice targets.

THE PLANNING PROCESS

Mission statement

The planning process is an iterative one, starting with the mission statement, or vision, of the organization. This needs to be meaningful to all members of the practice and have relevance to those others with an interest in the practice's success.

The mission statement answers the question 'Why do we exist?'. It, therefore, provides the *raison d'être* for the practice and:

- ◆ Describes the practice's identity.
- ◆ States the strategic objectives of the practice.
- ◆ Defines the services available from the practice.
- ◆ Is cautiously optimistic (realistic and believable).
- ◆ Arises from deeds and personal beliefs, not wishful thinking.
- ◆ Is clear to read and understand.
- ◆ Shows benefit to the practice, its patients and the health authority/health board.
- ◆ Is inspirational, answering the question 'Why would we be proud to work for this practice?'.

The following is an example from a practice:

> *To provide a comprehensive range of consistent high-quality primary health care services which are patient centred including effective drug therapy and access to secondary care services within a reasonable timeframe. To educate patients and stimulate an awareness in them of their own health needs and to use the resources of the NHS, particularly general medical services, in a responsible and appropriate manner.*

For practices wishing to develop a mission statement, a useful starting point could be the NHS mission statement.

The purpose of the NHS is to secure through the resources available the greatest possible improvement to the physical and mental health of the people of England by: promoting health, preventing ill-health, diagnosing and treating disease and injury, and caring for those with long-term illness and disability; a service available to all on the basis of clinical need, regardless of the ability to pay. In seeking to achieve this purpose, the NHS, as a public service, aims to judge its results under three headings – equity, efficiency and responsiveness.

Values and mission statement

The values which underpin the vision are equally important, because they embody the practice's ideals and offer a 'moral' or 'ethical' code to guide decision making. Some of these decisions are becoming increasingly difficult, as the NHS struggles with making the best use of available resources to improve the health of the population. This can sometimes be at variance with the best treatment for an individual patient, which is the traditional approach of doctors practising medicine. Having an explicit set of values can, therefore, be useful in communicating these difficult decisions to patients and others.

One practice has stated its values as a philosophy . . .

To provide the best possible care for our patients in a cost-effective way which is responsive to their needs. To maintain our commitment to a democratic way of practice with a tradition of easy access, team working and shared workload based on personal lists within a group practice.

To maintain and improve the standards of general medical practice by regular review, audit, education and the development of quality indicators.

To expand and develop practice services as much as is financially possible.

Environmental analysis

Once the practice has determined its vision or mission statement, and the values which guide it, the plan should reflect the external environment. This covers sociological, technological, economic and political factors which will influence the practice's survival. These are necessarily broad ranging and could include, for example, changes to the GP contract, the building of a new nursing home or housing estate, the closure of a local factory or a change in local or national government. The NHS as a whole has identified the following as key environmental factors – changing demographics, rising power of consumers and continuing developments in medical technology.

SWOT (strengths, weaknesses, opportunities and threats)

The SWOT analysis looks at the strengths, weaknesses, opportunities and threats relevant to the practice. This is a useful starting point in the planning process and concentrates on local factors. This includes the people (skills, training and development), the premises (information technology (IT), management and systems), service provision and development, quality, communication and management. It allows the practice to take an inventory of the skills and knowledge of the practice team – a useful exercise to develop ideas for the services which the practice could and should offer in the future.

The aim of the SWOT technique is to identify the extent to which the current strategy of an organization and its more specific strengths and weaknesses are relevant to, and capable of dealing with, changes taking place in the environment. So this technique looks at the key points for the practice which make it different from other practices or service providers in its area.

Ideally, this involves all members of the primary health care team and contributes to communication, teamwork and ownership of the planning process.

How is a SWOT constructed?

Strengths

These are internal to the practice and are those factors which give the practice advantage over others. They are, therefore, the key differences between the practice and other practices in the area. However, it may not be easy to identify these differences, so the list is likely to be based on perceptions. Boxes 4.3–4.6 show elements of a SWOT analysis.

Box 4.3
Strengths – example

1. Motivated, committed and enthusiastic staff.
2. Broad range of background experience.
3. Experienced practice/fundholding manager.

Weaknesses

These are also internal to the practice and may be skill shortages, resource problems or obstacles which have been identified.

Box 4.4
Weaknesses – example

1. Undeveloped IT system.
2. Duplicated/overlapping services between staff.
3. Unmodernized premises.

Opportunities

These are external developments which could enhance the practice's future position if taken advantage of. They are useful to identify future growth of service development. Getting these right can mean the difference between long-term practice survival and organizational decay.

Box 4.5
Opportunities –
example

> 1. Change to GP contract.
> 2. Primary care-led NHS initiative.
> 3. Expansion of purpose-built premises.
> 4. Setting up of an out-of-hours cooperative.

Threats

These are current or future developments which may affect the practice adversely. They need monitoring and dealing with, wherever possible.

Box 4.6
Threats – example

> 1. Lack of competition for secondary care services.
> 2. New partnership moving into area.
> 3. Loss of a partner.
> 4. Increasing administrative workload.

As well as creating the SWOT, a summary of reasons for good or poor practice performance is useful at this stage to put the proposed developments later in the plan into context. The SWOT should be condensed to the five or six key points under each of the headings. These will be the most important to tackle. It is also worth remembering that today's strengths can easily become tomorrow's weaknesses and vice versa. For example, a practice nurse with specialist skills may run the asthma clinic. The nurse may move away, leaving a requirement to find a replacement (see Box 4.7, p. 78).

Key issues These will emerge from the SWOT analysis. They are the factors which will have a high impact on future success for the practice. Some may be outside the practice's control. Where that is the case, it is sensible to adopt a 'watching brief' on them and see if, over time, they become factors about which something can be done. Other issues will be in areas where action needs to be taken and it is on these that efforts should be focused. Key issues should be expressed in the plan as statements or questions, otherwise they may simply repeat the bullet points outlined in the SWOT. Statements or questions will make setting the critical success factors, the next stage of the process, easier. By generating a handful of key issues the plan will emphasize those that are genuinely important. If the list ends up too long, it is unlikely that they can all be addressed effectively, when it comes to writing the action plans.

Some questions to ask when generating the list of key issues would be:

Box 4.7
SWOT check list

Questions to help generate the SWOT:

1. Internal:
   ◆ Which health care services are we best at? (taking into account the different areas of interest and expertise of the partners and staff)
   ◆ What are our outputs? (an output is a visible result of an action taken)
   ◆ What structure do we and should we have? (jobs, organization, functions)
   ◆ What internal and external communication systems do we have? (e.g. best use of IT links between the practice and the health authority/health board, and/ or hospital or community providers)
   ◆ What opportunities are there for new and/or improved services?
   ◆ What human resources do we need? (numbers, skills, competencies)
   ◆ What is our financial strength? (reserves, cashflow, margins)

2. External:
   ◆ Are there economic factors which may affect our ability to meet objectives?
   ◆ Are we aware of local environmental developments which may affect our activities?
   ◆ Have we considered the strengths and weaknesses of other practices in the area?

◆ Should any services be excluded entirely? If not, what priorities should be assigned to current service developments?
◆ Do clinical guidelines offer a suitable way forward to provide high-quality care?

Examples of a key issue are:

◆ How can we reduce unnecessary consultations?
◆ How can we develop the primary health care team? (based on the strength of 'breadth of staff experience', but the weakness of 'duplicated/overlapping services between staff')
◆ How can we balance high-quality medical care with cost constraints?

Critical success factors   These factors are those that must be addressed in order to achieve the objectives of the practice and answer the questions posed in the key issues section. The practice must perform well in order to achieve its objectives and live up to its mission statement, so the critical success factors are the major decision areas for the practice. The statements are best expressed as positive and action-orientated, in order to provide appropriate answers for the questions posed before. They should not be vague statements, because it is more difficult to recognize when the factor has been achieved. Critical success factors should consider what the practice needs to succeed today and in the future. For this to happen, there has to be balance in the practice's approach to managing its day-to-day business and to look at its future survival in the longer term.

Some questions to help in defining critical success factors are:

♦ What services must the practice provide to patients?
♦ How will we work with other agencies (trusts, health authorities and health boards, social services, etc.) to provide effective and appropriate care for patients?

Some examples of critical success factors are:

♦ Create clinical guidelines which will address patient needs in a cost-effective way (addressing the key issue of 'how can we balance high-quality medical care with cost constraints?').
♦ Increase the range of services available to patients, provided from the surgery (addressing the key issue of 'how can we develop the primary health care team?').
♦ Write a practice procedures manual (addressing the key issue of 'how can we reduce unnecessary consultations?').

OBJECTIVES Up to now, the plan has answered the question 'Where are we now?'. The second of the planning questions is 'Where do we want to be?'. The list of objectives will be the answer to this and follows from the SWOT, key issues and critical success factors. Objectives are usefully phrased as statements, in this case SMART (specific, measurable, agreed – and actionable, realistic and timebound) and will use action-oriented words. Objectives are expressed as ... 'To' ... 'help in making sure that something has to be *done* to achieve them'.

Examples are:

♦ To protect the existing in-house services and to continue to develop new services.
♦ To develop in-house consultant services (e.g. dermatology, audiology).
♦ To improve the internal management structure and development of clinical services.
♦ To improve and enhance information technology.
♦ To develop, over the next 12 months, and subsequently work within, guidelines for best clinical practice in x conditions.
♦ To extend disease management clinics to patients with asthma

and diabetes.

◆ To restart routine health visits to the elderly.

◆ To start hormone replacement therapy clinics and expand health promotion sessions.

Questions to be asked while developing objectives are shown in Box 4.8.

It is helpful to include costings, giving some idea of the resources

Box 4.8
Key questions in
setting objectives

◆ How realistic is this for us?

◆ How will we measure this?

◆ When should this be done by?

needed to achieve the objectives set. It is also important to list the assumptions made in deciding the objectives. It ensures progress towards them can be more accurately defined and any shortfall is likely to have an explanation. The assumptions explain the conditions under which the objectives are achievable. If they change, it will affect the practice's ability to deliver them.

ACTION PLANS   Having answered the question 'Where do we want to get to?', the third planning question is 'How do we get there?'. This is where the practice can start to consider the list of activities or inputs, which will define the responsibilities and accountabilities for achieving the objectives. These are the basis for the work plans for individuals in the practice and will help everyone to see where their contribution fits in to the practice's overall success. The action plans will also include more detail on the costings needed to undertake all the planned activities and will contribute to the practice budget.

The process associated with generating action plans can be broken down into seven steps (Box 4.9).

So far, the planning process has considered where the practice wants to be, through deciding where and how it wishes to develop and has put in place the milestones which will enable achievement of practice objectives.

Contingency   Although it is usual to write a plan which will deal with the most
planning   likely future scenario, it is a useful discipline to consider the question 'what if . . .' as well. In this way, the practice is less likely to be taken by surprise – pleasantly or unpleasantly. It is tempting to say 'we'll think about that if it happens', but that is a poor position for responding quickly and appropriately. It is helpful, then, to have an idea in advance, so that when the situation arises, the practice

Box 4.9
Formulation of an
action plan

1. Agree objectives and set targets with all those responsible for achieving them.
2. List all tasks and actions.
3. Agree individual responsibilities. It is important to allocate the responsibility for coordinating the plan – that person acts as the catalyst to ensure that everyone in the practice participates in the planning process.
4. Identify additional resources and skills required to achieve the plan (people, money, time).
5. Set a realistic timetable. This is helpful in keeping the plan moving forward.
6. Monitor and review progress. Too often, plans end up on shelves, dusty and unread. Regular review meetings are useful to ensure everyone is still working to the same plan. This part of the process answers the fourth planning question 'How far have we got?'.
7. Formal review and celebration. This will assess the impact of the plan and recognizes the significant contribution made by all in the practice team.

can capitalize on an opportunity or minimize the impact of a threat. For example, a fundholding practice may consider 'What if . . . our referrals budget runs out in month 9?'.

Risk management Another aspect of planning which it is easy to overlook is in dealing with risk. This is dealt with in more detail in another book in this series (the *Clinician's Management Handbook*) but it is useful to consider the types of risk which may require thought by the practice:

♦ Alleged clinical negligence is probably the most obvious type of risk facing a practice.
♦ Health and safety: this is an important consideration both for the practice staff and for the patients who visit the surgery.
♦ Documentation: this extends beyond the confidentiality of individual patient records, to consent forms for treatment, and the records for the building and equipment, staff contracts of employment, financial records, etc.

Plans for risk management should consider:

♦ Risk identification, look at what could go wrong and what the consequences might be.
♦ Risk analysis, taking the identified risk and deciding the incidence of it happening and its severity, and the associated costs.
♦ Risk control, either by avoiding the risk altogether, eliminating

it, minimizing the possibility of the risk occurring and the costs associated with it.

♦ Risk funding, often through insurance (e.g. MPS, MDU).

PLANNING TOOLS Some useful tools in creating the plan have already been described (SWOT analysis and the action plans process). There are other tools available to help with the planning process.

Forecasting This technique attempts to predict what the future would look like by extrapolating forward from historical trends. An example of this is the work done by Office of Population Censuses and Surveys (OPCS) in predicting the demographics of the UK population in the year 2010. It is this work that recognizes there will be fewer tax payers in the next decade and more elderly who will be relying on the NHS to provide them with good-quality health care. There are a number of IT packages which can assist in making this process easier. A simple combination of a spreadsheet and a graphics package (into which data can be imported) can be used to represent what has happened in the past and draw a best-fit extrapolation from the data presented. A number of alternatives can also be modelled, e.g. the impact of a new day case surgery unit opening in the locality. This would affect waiting list size and would also have an impact on the practice budget, with a different cost per procedure compared to the previous contract specification.

Decision making Often, the practice will need to consider where to invest and disinvest resources to deal with changes in the practice profile. A number of possible approaches can be taken to assist here. One of the most useful and simple to apply is modelled on the approach that *Which* magazine uses in comparisons of different products. The principle is that a number of products or services are all considered against the same set of criteria and the option which scores highest wins. In planning health services, some authorities have adopted this approach and it should work as well for individual practices.

One example is given here. The authority identified criteria which reflected values of the organization. Each of these criteria were weighted as shown in Figure 4.3.

Having decided on the set of criteria against which all proposals would be considered, the authority allocated up to 10 points for each option against each criteria, giving a possible maximum of 1000 points. In this way, the authority was able to determine which proposals would be suitable for investment. In the same way, the proposals which scored least against these criteria could be areas for disinvestment (Figure 4.4).

Figure 4.3
Methodology for
selecting and
prioritizing proposals
for investing in health
care gain

Criteria	Weighting
Potential for health gain	40
Potential for improved quality of service	20
Accordance with local view	20
Achievability	15
Accordance with national priorities	5

Source: Wandsworth Health Authority (1991) in Honigsbaum *et al*. (1995).

Factors and values	Potential for health gain	Improved quality of service	Accordance with local view	Achievability	Accordance with national priorities	Total
	40	20	20	15	5	
Option 1						
Option 2						
Option 3						
Option 4						
Option 5						
Option 6						

Figure 4.4
Option appraisal for alternative services

ORGANIZATIONAL NEEDS AND REQUIREMENTS In considering the planning process, the resources identified will be partly responsible for ensuring the success or failure of the plan. These are defined in terms of people, money, time and IT. If resources are used appropriately, the chances of the plan's success improve. The management of people, finance and IT are dealt with in some depth in other chapters. However, it is worth looking briefly at the 'stakeholder' aspect of managing people.

People The most important resource for the practice is its people. In addition to the members of the practice team, there are others, who are the people who will ultimately judge the success or failure of the plan. They are either concerned with the role they play in implementing parts of the plan or are likely to benefit from the proposals made in the plan. It is, therefore, important to recognize who these people are and to ensure that they are involved to an appropriate degree in the generation and/or implementation of the plan. So, in planning the timetable for the generation of the plan and identifying timescales for the action plans to be carried out, it is useful to build in time, not just for the tasks to be done, but to obtain the commitment necessary from these different groups. This is the process of 'managing stakeholders' and their expectations.

Useful questions at this point are:

♦ Who wants us to succeed, and why?
♦ Who will be affected by our success or failure and in what way?
♦ Who do we need to be involved in our plan?
♦ What are the costs and benefits to them of involvement?
♦ What could they do to prevent success of the plan?

By addressing their specific areas of interest or concern and making use of any special expertise they may have, the chances of success for the plan will be improved. In this way the contribution of the following groups can be considered – practice staff, patients, the health authority or health board, trusts and other suppliers to the practice of products and services, local patient support groups, the Community Health Council (CHC), social services, education, housing and voluntary groups.

The job of the planning coordinator is to fit the reality of the plan to the measures of success that each of these groups will expect the plan to deliver. For example, there will be those who will expect to be informed of any changes prior to the change occurring, others who need to be informed as the change happens and those who will only need to be informed once the change has been put in place. It is the experience of many organizations that it is this part of the process, managing stakeholders, which may be most easily overlooked and so is worth significant attention.

IDENTIFYING PERFORMANCE OR QUALITY INDICATORS   By paying special attention to the requirements of stakeholders, a number of the key measures of success are identified which need to be included in the plan. These will be part of the performance indicators and quality measures which need to be reported against in the annual report, in addition to the requirements laid down in legislation.

Measures of health, illness and patient satisfaction are essential to the establishment of needs for and outcomes of health care. (Wilkin *et al.*, 1992)

The following list considers a number of top-line quality indicators which can be used by the practice to determine whether practice activity, in cooperation with other services provided for patients, will generate improvements in health status over time. For example, morbidity targets may look at reduction in incidence or prevalence, minimization of the effects of disease or symptom control (as measured in chronic disease management clinics), absence, reversal or stabilization of disease.

Box 4.10
Quality indicators

◆ Mortality:
  − Reduction in mortality from a given condition
  − Reduction in avoidable deaths
  − Increase in life expectancy

◆ Morbidity:
  − Reduction in incidence
  − Reduction in prevalence
  − Reduction in preventable ill-health
  − Minimization of the effects of disease/symptom control
  − Absence of disease
  − Reversal or stabilization of disease

◆ Physical function:
  − Ability to feed oneself
  − Improved ambulation
  − Ability to dress oneself
  − Ability to bathe oneself

◆ Psychological function:
  − Reduction in anxiety
  − Acceptance of death (terminal care)

◆ Unplanned use of care:
  − Reduction in re-admissions to hospital
  − Reduction in complication rates
  − Reduction in prolonged, lengthy stays in hospital
  − Reduction in prolonged courses of treatment

◆ Occupational functions:
  − Decrease in days off work/school because of poor control of condition

◆ Health-related knowledge and behaviour:
  − Increased understanding by patients of condition
  − Increased compliance with treatment
  − More lifestyle advice given
  − Changed behaviour patterns (e.g. reduced alcohol/ tobacco consumption, increased exercise, diet changes)

◆ Patient satisfaction:
  − Increased access to services
  − Increased convenience (e.g. changed appointment system)
  − Increased perception of quality
  − Increased equality in response to equal need

It is these areas which will demonstrate health gain and improvements to the services offered to the practice patients.

MEASURING
TECHNIQUES
The indicators can be measured using a variety of techniques. Each of these evaluation techniques can provide useful feedback to the practice about the services it provides, or commissions for patients. Taking each in turn, starting with a useful, but subjective method.

Anecdotal evidence
This, by itself, is not particularly useful, as one anecdote can be countered by another. However, it can be a useful sanity check to confirm or refute information provided by other methods. Making a collection of anecdotes and then applying judgement can be useful to increase the robustness of the anecdotal findings. It is interesting to note that this form of evaluation is sometimes given greater credence than is warranted considering the subjectivity of the measure.

Complaints and
compliments
1996 saw the introduction of new complaints procedures in general practice, health authorities, health boards and trusts. Patients are encouraged to complain through these channels and it will be interesting to see whether the national culture (which is not, traditionally, a complaining one) will embrace this system. More often, at least as far as the health service goes, patients are likely to compliment service providers, and general practice in particular, for the job they do. The Patients Charter has given patients a platform against which to judge services and this enables them to determine when a complaint may be made. The 'in-house' mechanism of dealing with complaints initially provides a means of measuring quality of service as well as resolving problems locally.

Case studies
This involves a staff member shadowing a patient through an episode of treatment and collecting their views, together with those of relatives or carers, staff and clinicians involved in the patient's management. The results are used to make recommendations for changes to the way in which the patient is treated, and to existing protocols.

In-depth patient
interviews
This can be used for patients with chronic diseases, or where the treatment is complex, perhaps involving more than one specialty. Again the results can be used to inform the contracting process and suggesting quality improvements which can be made to patient care.

Patient surveys
These can be employed either to assess treatment which has been provided or to collect suggestions on how treatment can be improved in the future. This provides a more quantifiable result than the methods suggested above. The results should be used in conjunction with the more subjective observations taken from the other techniques. Patient satisfaction is a subjective evaluation of physical and mental well-being, but is a valid part of evaluating

treatments – perception is all. Among the factors which might influence feelings of satisfaction are:

◆ Outcome of treatment/care received.
◆ Staff approach and attitudes.
◆ Quality of information on what to do and what to expect.
◆ Appointment procedures.
◆ Waiting times.
◆ General facilities available.
◆ For in-patients, 'hotel' facilities (e.g. quality of food, privacy, visiting arrangements).

Audit   This provides a systematic process for measuring outputs in terms of improved (or otherwise) patient outcomes. It considers the quality of medical care, including the procedures for diagnosis and treatment, the use of resources and the resulting outcome and quality of life for the patient. As audit is one of the activities in which practices should be participating, it is appropriate to consider it in more detail here.

The seven-step audit approach has been used successfully in different aspects of health care audit, whether in general practice, hospitals, for unidisciplinary or multidisciplinary audit. The seven steps form a logical process to measure the success of health service interventions and make some judgement about whether the service under investigation represents a good use of health service resources.

Seven-step audit approach

1. Design the audit (selecting the subjects suitable for audit, clarifying the audit objectives, assigning staff responsibilities and selecting the patients).
2. Decide criteria and agree standards (see the list of quality indicators above).
3. Collect and organize data (e.g. screening patient notes against the indicators can be done either manually or by computer, and will give a snapshot of current practice performance in terms of processes and outcomes).
4. Analyse audit data. This should show where the processes and outcomes do not meet the quality indicators or, indeed, the clinical needs of the patients.
5. Identify cause of non-achievement. This is the part of the process which diagnoses the reasons for non-achievement and enables the practice to consider what changes are required.
6. Implement changes (using the action plan process and managing stakeholders approach).
7. Monitor progress. This will establish whether the action plan correctly addresses the problem identified in step 5. If not, a

different action plan may need to be generated, or different timescales assigned to put the audit back on track.

In order for audit to provide a fundamental building block in measuring the performance of the practice team, it is focused on the needs of the patient and the practice, and can usefully identify where changes should be made, e.g. in setting up and using clinical guidelines, in rewriting contracts with secondary care providers, or in making changes within the practice.

Research   This can be particularly useful where a new or experimental procedure is planned. Provision has been made for fundholding practices to use any savings in research which increases the scope for robust information to be generated about the services which are provided for patients in primary care and community settings.

OTHER PERFORMANCE INDICATORS   In addition to the quality measures discussed above, there are other, more management orientated methods to monitor the performance of the practice. Some of these are covered in the requirements for the content of the annual report:

◆ List size.
◆ Age/sex register.
◆ Consultation rates.
◆ Out-of-hours visits.
◆ Hospital referrals (inpatient, outpatient, day case, including self-referrals, where known).
◆ Minor surgery arrangements.
◆ Preventative care, e.g. immunizations, vaccinations, cervical cytology, health promotion and disease management clinics.
◆ Disease register (infectious and notifiable diseases, malignant neoplasms, diseases of the circulatory system, asthma, diabetes, epilepsy, coronary heart disease).
◆ Use of clinical guidelines or formulary arrangements.

The structure of the practice itself can generate useful additional information if compared with other practices in the area, providing a similar range of services. It can also help in defining the work plan for the practice team, as described later:

◆ The number of staff, other than doctors, assisting the doctor in his or her practice, including total numbers, their principal duties and hours worked each week, their qualifications and any training they have undertaken in the past 5 years.
◆ Premises information, including variations in floor space, design or quality over the past year, or planned during the next 12 months.
◆ The doctors' other commitments as a medical practitioner in terms of posts held, work undertaken and time involved.

Management by In considering the measurement of individuals working within the
objectives practice, management by objectives is a useful technique which fits
well with the planning process. The plan itself provides the framework against which individuals' contributions can be defined and
measured (Glaxo Wellcome, 1996).

The steps involved in management by objectives are:

1. Specify performance requirements.
2. Design jobs and functions.
3. Develop practice capability and culture.
4. Develop staff.
5. Provide rewards.

Management using this system gives responsibility to individuals
within the practice to monitor their progress, both individually and
collectively against the requirements of the plan. The practice
should support this, with development programmes for practice
staff, recognition and celebration when objectives have been
achieved and, of course, ensuring that the plan is understood by
the whole practice. This area is covered in some detail, in the
chapter on human resource management.

CONCLUSION The current health care environment requires that general practice, incorporating the wider primary care team, is run as a cost-
effective business, in line with all other commercial and service
organizations. This involves starting with a corporate or business
plan of what needs to be achieved, and more importantly, what the
practice wants to achieve in order to be proactive. The alternative
is to be purely market led, responding to government or health
authority bureaucracy.

The constraints of general practice are always time- and patient-
driven demands. However, these pressures can be controlled
through proactive planning, and by identifying and planning for
development in primary care before they hit the practice. Practices
are already responding to this challenge through GP consortia and
out of hours cooperatives, but more work could be done in this
process, in the form of improved business planning.

Although staff form approximately 70% of total management
costs and are, therefore, an expensive resource, they are often
overlooked in drawing up the plans to which they must be
committed. Successful business planning relies on realistically
formulated plans, but relies equally on motivated staff who will
contribute to, share and implement the 'vision' of the practice in
order to ensure its long-term survival.

The planning measures advocated in this chapter may at first
seem to be time consuming and resource intensive, but there is
truth in the adage 'to invest in time is to save time'. The time

investment required will lead to greater control of both external and internal pressures, and less firefighting.

At a time when primary care initiatives can seize the health care agenda, strategic and operational planning are absolutely crucial for success.

SUMMARY

♦ Planning is a continuous process to improve the quality of care for patients and defines the organizational requirements needed to deliver such improvements.

♦ The plan enables the practice to identify where changes in working practices will generate these quality improvements year on year, towards a health gain goal for patients.

♦ The plan defines the roles and responsibilities of all practice staff and other stakeholders in achieving the objectives for the practice and, by doing so, will improve the quality of working life for the practice team.

♦ The plan allows the practice to identify and bid for additional resources needed to deliver health gain objectives, which will take into account the variations between each practice and others in the area.

♦ The plan provides a focus and identity for the members of the practice team and a recognition that all are involved in achievement of the plan's objectives.

FURTHER READING

♦ Burns, P., Harrison, J. (1992). Business planning made easy. How to chart your way ahead. *Medeconomics* 1(10): 20.

♦ Campbell, A. (1991). Business Planning – a boost for GPs. *Medeconomics* 12(12): 47.

♦ Hansell, D.M. and Salter, B. (1995). *The Clinician's Management Handbook*. W.B. Saunders, London.

♦ The National Health Service (General Medical and Pharmaceutical Services) Regulations, (1989), Schedule 1L, regulation 3 (2) SI (1597). Department of Health, London.

♦ Roberts, H. (1990). *Outcome and Performance in Healthcare*. Public Finance Foundation, London.

♦ Warren, C. (1993). Business plans put you in the fast lane. *Medeconomics* 9 January: 37.

♦ Wilkin, D., Hallam, K. and Doggett, M.A. (1992). *Measures of Need and Outcome for Primary Health Care*. Oxford University Press, Oxford.

REFERENCES   Glaxo Wellcome UK Ltd (1996), *Progressive Practice*.

Honigsbaum, F., Calltorp, J., Ham, C. and Holstrom, S. *Priority Setting Processes for Healthcare*. Radcliffe Medical Press, Oxford.

Roe, P. and Semple Piggot, C. (1994), *Health Gain and How to Achieve it.* Glaxo Pharmaceuticals UK Ltd, London.

Semple Piggot, C. (1996), *Business Planning for NHS Managers*. Kogan Page, London.

Wilkin, D., Hallam, K. and Doggett, M.A. (1992), *Measures of Need and Outcome for Primary Health Care*. Oxford University Press, Oxford.

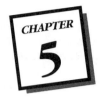

NEGOTIATION IN MANAGEMENT

CHAPTER 5

Claire Hill

OBJECTIVES

♦ To identify areas where general practice requires sound negotiation techniques in both its provider and purchaser roles.

♦ To explore and explain the knowledge and skills needed to maximize a satisfactory outcome.

♦ To examine the two vital components in a successful negotiation, i.e. interpersonal skills and procedural conventions.

♦ To describe techniques of negotiation at a team and an individual level.

♦ To identify the competitive advantage afforded by the above.

INTRODUCTION

Negotiation skills are part of the essential tool kit for everyday life and are practised automatically over workloads, deadlines and contracts. They are particularly important where it is necessary to persuade others to do things that they feel perhaps unwilling or unable to do, even over mundane issues such as the allocation of chores, or how late the children stay up or what they can watch on television.

It is now vital for general practitioners (GPs) to understand and practise the procedures and skills employed by the best negotiators, in order to maximize success in the internal market created in the 1990s. The fundholding model will evolve and change, but contracting for health in a managed market is the rapidly developing model of the future. The contracting process will be controlled increasingly by GP purchasing and indeed by new provider opportunities. However, it must be recognized that, as a result of the doctor–patient consultation itself, many GPs will already regard themselves as experienced negotiators! The consultation process of eliciting evidence and facts, weighing up options and reaching a negotiated outcome is a skill shared by many members of the primary health care team. Indeed, the best medical receptionists, coping with the 'front-line' problems will be very good negotiators.

This is, therefore, no new management jargon in general practice, but such abilities are not inherent. No one is a born negotiator, but everyone can learn and practise tried and tested methods to turn him or her into more effective negotiators. There is never a shortage of situations in which to practise these skills, and they will contribute to less stress and a better quality of life, both at work and at home. Unfortunately, they are most likely to be forgotten in those personally stressful situations when they are most needed! This can be countered by a better understanding of interpersonal skills and processes both in ourselves and in others.

There is virtually no gain in learning the conventions of good negotiation without an understanding of the interpersonal skills needed to make the conventions work. Similarities may be drawn here to a game of chess. Simply learning the conventions of the moves is only the first step in fully understanding how to win the game.

This chapter will explore both aspects to enable practitioners to win the game as often as possible.

WHAT IS NEGOTIATION? Negotiation is a way of reaching agreement without having to impose your will over somebody else or giving in to another person's demands.

Certain situations or decisions are of course non-negotiable, but there are many other occasions where the ability to persuade others of the merits of your way of thinking, or of a service you are offering, will achieve a superior and more satisfactory outcome. The most successful result is usually where both parties feel at least reasonably satisfied, particularly where the relationship is ongoing, such as with your partner or spouse!

WHY NEGOTIATE? The importance of effective negotiation techniques and strategies is widely underestimated. The value of acquiring the skills and knowledge of the processes are two-fold:

- ◆ Personal effectiveness. It enhances personal effectiveness, self-esteem and confidence in knowing that you have a 'tool kit' to handle potentially difficult situations involving a conflict of interest or opinion, whether this be with the health authority, a hospital consultant or your bank manager.
- ◆ Business advantage. The value lies in knowing that such a tool kit translates into business advantages which are tangible and measurable.

The principle is always to achieve low-cost, high-value outcomes, although the value often lies in a personal advantage, and not always one with a financial price attached to it. In a business environment, this reflects a culture which has been alien to the National Health Service (NHS), but the internal market makes it essential for practitioners to be able to maximize the potential of the practice in the purchasing or marketing of services, and in the use of resources.

This chapter is essentially about how to resolve differences to the best advantage. Such advantages will often be personal, but could apply equally to a situation where you are asked for advice by one party in a difference of opinion with another, or where you are between the two parties in disagreement, both of which situations occur occasionally in all work environments.

Negotiation skills in all these situations can be learned with application and practice. They are dealt with and explored in two sections (Box 5.1).

Box 5.1
Negotiation skills

♦ Communication, persuasion and conflict-resolution skills.

♦ Tactical and procedural skills during the stages of a negotiation.

WHAT ARE THE SKILLS AND THE ADVANTAGES?

Persuasion

The ability to persuade others to see a different point of view which is more advantageous to yourself. However, this is not a one-sided transaction. It involves a genuine ability to listen to and understand conflicting or alternative points of view. Other people can only be won over if they feel their view is genuinely considered and understood. Everyone has suffered the experience of putting their views across to people whom, they know, might be giving the appearance of listening but then take no account of what has been said, usually because they have been rehearsing a counterargument and giving only partial attention to the speaker. Such tactics rarely achieve any advantages in negotiation but, rather, lead to an aggravation of the situation.

Conflict resolution

Negotiation skills are essential in the art of conflict resolution. Conflict can range from a latent, unvoiced form, to a manifest display of anger, but whether it is suppressed or bursts out (and there are clearly many stages on the continuum), it is distressingly disruptive to team spirit and the harmonious running of the practice. Most of our energies are dedicated to avoiding conflict instead of confronting it in a constructive, positive way. Conflict avoidance sows the seeds of discontent, usually leading to problems escalating, but rarely disappearing.

People often work together for years, devoting time to covering up carefully causes of disagreement and potential conflict instead of channelling the same energies into dealing with them. This is dangerous because, at best, it impairs working relationships and destroys underlying trust and honesty. At worst, a relatively small matter of disagreement can escalate into a 'last straw' situation, and cause a heated exchange or outburst which both parties find subsequently uncomfortable and difficult to deal with, leading to further withdrawal from the person and the problem.

This is a situation with which GPs will be familiar, either from first-hand experiences or hearing about it from colleagues. It is a contributing factor to GPs leaving to join other practices and is one of the best reasons to incorporate conflict-resolution skills as part of your negotiating tool kit.

Confidence   Acquiring negotiation skills and the knowledge of how to use them provide an enormous confidence boost, just through knowing that you can face and deal with an uncomfortable situation, and just as importantly, enable the other party to do the same. Such attributes are quickly recognized and valued by those around you, and the same skills used in resolution of personal conflicts will be in demand in other areas, e.g. in resolving long-standing, perhaps unspoken conflict between partners, or receptionists, or in difficult negotiations with the health authority or a provider of services.

The three main advantages of negotiation skills are therefore:

Box 5.2
Advantages of
negotiation skills

> ♦ Persuasion – the ability to persuade others to see a different point of view.
>
> ♦ Conflict resolution – avoiding conflict sows the seeds of discontent leading to escalation of the problem.
>
> ♦ Confidence – knowing you can face and deal with an uncomfortable situation which others will avoid.

THE IMPORTANCE OF THE WIN–WIN OR 'FEEL-GOOD' FACTOR   It helps in obtaining an effective advantage in any negotiation, to recognize the importance of the 'feel-good' factor in the other party. If the cost of your 'winning' (whether it be a moral or financial victory) leaves the other party feeling devalued or the 'loser', subsequent communications or gaining any further advantages will certainly be a lot more difficult and may prove impossible.

If as much energy is devoted to thinking through the other party's needs as your own and in identifying how you could go some way to satisfying his or her personal agenda (and you may well need to look outside the scope of the immediate issue), then you will be well on the way to achieving what is called a 'win–win' situation. This is a situation where you need to have achieved the best result you can, but one in which the other party also feels he or she has won something of value.

The cause of failure in a negotiating situation is often because we think through carefully what we want to achieve, whilst not fully taking into account the needs of the other person.

Figure 5.1 gives an example in the primary care team of a potential conflict which is in danger of focusing on matters such as roles and positions instead of reconciling any mutal interests. It demonstrates totally different outcomes, depending on the negotiation stance adopted. Whilst the first scenario results in a nurse who feels undervalued and may look for alternative employment opportunities, the second scenario results in a mutually satisfactory compromise. It should be remembered that the outcome of such a

---

Take, for example, a 'territorial' or delegation conflict in general practice:

> A new practice nurse has just been taken on. Previously only the GPs have undertaken cervical cytology but the nurse wishes this procedure to be part of her professional responsibilities. She states her strongly held position that she should develop this area of expertise. The senior partner states categorically the practice's position – that only doctors undertake such potentially difficult procedures because of the risks involved.

↓

The result of this exchange?

> Impasse, achieving a 'win–lose' situation whereby the senior partner might feel satisfied, but the nurse certainly will not. This focuses on positions instead of interests.

Focusing on interests, the exchange could have taken the following format:

> The practice nurse discusses that she would like to maximize her contribution to patient care teamwork through undertaking cervical cytology and, in doing so, further her professional expertise whilst relieving the partners of some of their current workload. Her interests are both personal career development and, potentially, those of the partners who need more time.

↓

The result is:

> The senior partner advises her that, whilst this has been regarded as a clinical responsibility for very good reasons, and would remain so, training and subsequent supervision could be undertaken, with a view to rethinking the situation after careful monitoring during a 12-month period.

The latter scenario is most likely to achieve a 'win–win' situation. Mutual interests are not always explicit, but will be sought and identified by an experienced negotiator.

Source: *Progress in Practice, Unit 7: Effective negotiation*, for Astra Pharmaceuticals, pp. 6–10, 14–16, reproduced with permission from Kluwer Academic Publishers, Lancaster, UK.

Figure 5.1
An example of negotiation.

situation will usually affect the morale and motivation of other team members.

THE ROLE OF COMMUNICATION IN EFFECTIVE NEGOTIATION

People recognise the need to communicate but find it difficult. Like Schopenhauer's hedgehogs, they want to get together, it's only their prickles that keep them apart. (Armstrong)

The most essential item in the armoury of a negotiator is good communication skills because issues are often complex, involve conflicting interests and can be emotionally testing. This section looks specifically at the role of communication in achieving success through influencing others and examines the key skills described in the first section.

Active listening

Active listening is about getting in touch with feelings; understanding your own and empathizing with the other person's. Issues commonly centre around opinions, facts and individual (often conflicting) positions, making it difficult to get to grips with the real underlying barriers to communication which are to do with feelings. Feelings are not always rational, and where there is a potential for differences of opinion, an understanding of the irrational is essential.

Active listening has to be practised to be acquired because, if you have a strongly held point of view, the temptation is to voice it before or without fully listening to a counteropinion. It involves self-restraint in listening to and, more importantly, understanding the other person's point of view before asserting your own.

Tuning into feelings is not commonly regarded as a British attribute and particularly not in a workplace. GPs are adept at tuning into patients' feelings, but their training and the nature of the profession make it more difficult to deal with their own feelings and those of partners and other members of the team.

Active listening is essentially about tuning into the feelings behind the words, or listening to what the person means, which may not be the same as what they say. The next step is to discover what motivates them to feel this way or to hold strong views which might be contrary to your own. These are similar skills to those required in coaching or counselling. Empathy is the key to active listening; demonstrating that you understand what they feel strongly about and why they feel this way. It is no coincidence that major corporations have promoted a listening image to customers. An example of this is the 'listening bank'. This is not pure altruism but translates into a business advantage.

An illustration of the importance of active listening is in staff negotiations. Changes which are put forward after detailed rational thought are never received in a rational way, if they involve changes to existing staffing arrangements. The following scenarios (Boxes 5.3–5.5) illustrate this point.

Box 5.3
Staffing negotiations for a new practice nurse

This involves separate sets of negotiations with partners, the health authority, and with existing staff on new or changed roles. The health authority part of the negotiation might be the most straightforward, if bureaucratically frustrating, so long as a supporting business plan exists, together with relevant job description(s) and a clear case is made based on patient population and practice activity. The more difficult negotiation is likely to be with existing staff on new or revised roles and responsibilities which constitute a real, potential or imagined threat to staff and perhaps to a partner.

Box 5.4
Staff negotiations to revise contracts

Occasionally the need will arise to amend or update staff contracts. This may be due to changes dictated by new employment law (e.g. when the same employment protection rights were afforded to part-time as for full-time staff), or may be part of a decision to tighten up or improve on procedures such as discipline or grievance, which should form part of the contract of employment. As in the previous scenario, the immediate staff reaction is likely to be hostile because of the perceived threat factor.

Box 5.5
Negotiations to merge nursing roles

In order to provide a more effective nursing resource based at practice level, an objective may be to merge the roles of the practice nurse, district nurse and health visitor. Their functional delineations may be regarded as no longer appropriate to modern general practice, and to impede flexibility on issues such as cover and providing seamless patient care. The word 'objective' rather than 'decision' was used carefully, because a decision represents a *fait accompli*, which makes a negotiation impossible and forces the parties into entrenched positions from which it is impossible to escape. This set of negotiations, involving changes to roles and perceived status, is likely to be the most difficult and protracted.

The scenarios described will be familiar to some extent to all those who are experienced in primary care management. *The barriers* to achieving your objectives in the above situations are:

♦ Focusing on your own position and status without understanding fully the similar needs of others.
♦ Not understanding the personal threat and real fear which your changes represent to those affected (whether real or imaginary).
♦ Not appreciating and properly preparing areas of common ground or mutual interests which can be used to build a constructive negotiation, leading to your desired outcome.

The successful outcome is achieved through:

♦ Sowing the seeds of change and enabling staff to feel they are contributing to the shape of things to come, i.e. things are not predetermined but subject to team input.
♦ Appreciating that change is potentially stressful to all staff, particularly when involving perceived status, position, salary or job security.
♦ Using active listening techniques to overcome barriers. Conflict is defused when it is clear that you are genuinely listening to the words and empathizing with the feelings. This enables rational argument to take place. The alternative to active listening is stating positions instead of building on mutual interests. The former never leads to a successful outcome.

Non-verbal communication or body language

Communication is not only about words and feelings, it also involves non-verbal communication or body language. It is estimated that at least 50% of all communication is conducted on a non-verbal level, which is why it is particularly important to learn the art of what people mean, not what they say. Body language often shows underlying irritation or discomfort which words belie.

For example, someone concealing true feelings or telling a lie will usually avoid direct eye contact or pass their hands over their mouth as they speak. In negotiations we do not always mean what we say. However, it is important that body language remains controlled and relaxed in order that it does not betray underlying concerns which contradicts words. In conclusion, the three levels of active listening can be portrayed as shown in Figure 5.2.

Persuasion and conflict-resolution skills

Ultimately ... conflict lies not in objective reality but in people's heads. (Fisher and Ury, 1983)

Handling a complaint or receiving personal criticism, or dealing with aggression is not easy for anyone. Immediate and natural defence barriers go up, often accompanied by feelings of irritation or indignant anger. Defensive behaviour is a natural but ill-thought-out reaction. It will lead to increased aggression in the other person, making the situation almost impossible to resolve. The

Figure 5.2
The three levels of
active listening

Source: *Progress in
Practice, Unit 7: Effective
negotiation*, for Asta
Pharmaceuticals, pp. 6–
10, 14–16, reproduced
with permission from
Kluwer Academic
Publishers, Lancaster, UK.

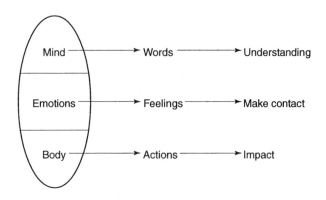

most effective technique is to listen without interruption to let the
other party let off steam, resisting the temptation to interject with
counterarguments (Box 5.6). Then briefly summarize your perception of how they feel. This will usually defuse all but the most
heated of complainants. After that, you should concentrate on facts
and issues, avoiding opinions or allowing any personality factors to
enter the discussion.

Box 5.6
Techniques of
resolving conflicts

- ◆ Listen without interruption.
- ◆ Summarize your perceptions.
- ◆ Concentrate on facts and issues.
- ◆ Avoid opinions and personality factors.

Where the hostility takes a personal form, this is the more
difficult and upsetting situation, which is most likely to induce a
defensive reaction. An effective technique in dealing with this is to
tell the other person calmly how you feel about what they said: 'I
feel very disappointed/upset at what you have said and that you
should feel that way, but I think it is important/good that we are
talking about it'.

Occasionally, of course, it can be beneficial to 'clear the air' in a
less controlled way but only if you can be certain it will clear the air
and that the outcome will not be worse. There normally has to be a
good existing relationship for two people to be able to have heated
arguments 'safely'. Expressing feelings is usually only an effective
technique if they are expressed in a calm and controlled way.

An often preferred alternative to dealing with the conflict is to
try to avoid it: to be passive or appeasing or to walk away from it.
The disadvantages of this approach are that the source of conflict

Figure 5.3
Checklist of areas that
may need attention

	Satisfactory performance	Some attention needed area	Key development area
Handling conflict in a priority or territory clash			
Broaching a difficult subject			
Disagreeing on a professional issue with a work colleague			
Handling a complaint and dealing with aggression			
Making a complaint			
Changing someone's mind – bringing them round to your way of thinking			
Saying 'No' assertively and positively			

does not disappear and covert conflict can be extremely divisive to working relationships. You have also failed to make your views and feelings understood. This denies the validity of your point of view and will usually be perceived by others as a weakness.

An action checklist to indicate areas of conflict which may need attention is a useful tool. An example is given in Figure 5.3.

STAGES AND STRATEGIES IN THE NEGOTIATION PROCESS

This section looks at the stages or conventions in negotiation, and at the strategies and styles most likely to bring success. The two commonly perceived and used approaches are that of the hard bargainer (who is tough and drives a hard deal making few concessions) and that of the soft bargainer (who seeks to avoid personal conflict and gives away more than is necessary).

However, there is a third approach, known as *principled negotiation* developed at the Harvard Negotiation Project. This method seeks mutual gains through focusing on interests, not positions. The advantage of this approach to negotiation is illustrated by the cervical cytology example in the last section. Guiding principles are to obtain low-cost, high-value solutions through being *hard on the issues but soft on the people*. It also introduces the more creative concept of developing a BATNA (best alternative to a negotiated agreement), which could be more advantageous than the traditional 'bottom line'.

Firstly, the stages and what they involve are explained, with particular emphasis paid to preparation, which is the single most important factor for a successful negotiation, and then strategies are explored.

Advance preparation

Research has demonstrated that preparation is the most consistent guide to negotiating performance. This involves identifying in advance:

♦ What you would ideally like to gain, i.e. best possible outcome.
♦ What you need to gain or must get.
♦ What you intend to gain.

This has been illustrated by the analogy of a hot-air balloonist planning his flight between London and Paris. He defined his objectives as follows:

> *I would* like *to make it to Paris in one hop but I certainly* intend *to land in France. At all costs I* must *avoid landing in the Channel.*

Preparation should take the form of a few headings, such as, objectives, information, concessions, strategy and tasks.

Objectives

Establish objectives and prioritize them realistically. All of them must be achievable, but some will carry more importance than others. Equally, think about the opposition's objectives and how these might be prioritized. If each party's objectives are all tablets of stone and each party is waiting for the other to move ground, it will be a long and unproductive meeting.

Information

This is essential for setting objectives. Without adequate information about relevant factors (e.g., the market, competition, financial opportunities or constraints), you are negotiating in a vacuum. Just as important is intelligence gathering on the other party. Information is the key to making informed assumptions about the opponent's objectives and priorities.

An example of this is fundholding budget negotiations with the health authority (HA). The fundholding budget originally set by the HA may be too low (the irony being that the more efficient the practice, the lower the budget was likely to be set). If the practice realizes that its budget was set too low, it will need up-to-date, detailed and relevant information to demonstrate this fact based on evidence of particular factors affecting its patient population. In some areas in particular, this could be higher than average deprivation levels, or a higher than average percentage of elderly and dependent people.

The HA criteria and opposition to any such argument needs to be researched, anticipated and countered before negotiations for the revised budget are commenced. This strategy is essential always to maximize the chances of a successful outcome, and is particularly important at times when HAs are seeking to reduce budgets still further.

The analogy of researching thoroughly factors which affect your budget apply equally outside the work situation.

To take a simple example, if you decide to buy a new car, you would not normally make the purchase before assessing the state of the market, e.g. new car sales are down in a recession, therefore, the salesman will be anxious to secure a deal and you should be in a strong negotiating position. Furthermore, your information tells you that you are likely to get £500 more for your present model by a private sale, but you estimate that, for the salesman, paying over the odds on a trade-in price is worth it to clinch the deal and achieve his (diminished) commission and target. You have found out that a rival main dealer offers free installation of an electronic sun roof on every new car purchased. You bring this information to light just before the salesman gets you to sign the sales agreement. Whilst he cannot move to the sun roof, he is prepared to throw in some further concessions which are of low cost to him, but represent high value to you, such as more favourable terms for a loan agreement.

It is a truism that information equals power. The more information you have about your own and your opponent's case, the better you are able to control negotiations. You then have to decide how much information revealed during the course of negotiations will further your progress. Information is powerful because it can structure the expected outcomes of your opponent. A selected filtering is, therefore, advantageous rather than full and open disclosure. This should be carefully thought through in advance and not left to intuition at the time.

Concessions and strategy

Strategy is similar to a game of chess, in that the grand plan, objectives and the opening moves need to be mapped out in advance, but great flexibility is required throughout. Strategy normally concentrates on the differences between the two sides, but should concentrate on establishing common interests, and from there common ground on which to build. It needs to take into account potential areas of conflict and how to counter these if and when they arise, building on the skills explained in the last section.

Almost always something has to be conceded for a mutually satisfactory negotiation. It is advisable to identify some concessions in advance (concessions which may even have been 'built in' to your side for this very purpose). This is part of the objective and priority-setting which is the first part of preparation. What might seem like a game is, in fact, an important ritual, e.g. if you decide to put your house on the market and the first potential buyer offers the full asking price, you will be left mildly dissatisfied. Should you have asked for more? Did you undersell yourself? This is part of the bargaining ritual, whereby both parties need to achieve a win–win outcome and feel satisfied.

The value of team roles in a negotiation

Tasks or roles

In the majority of normal negotiation situations, we act as an individual but some more important negotiations may be conducted with a partner or with a professional grouping. In this situation, as much attention needs to be directed to the roles of the 'home team' as to the opposition.

Any division in the ranks (often expressed unconsciously in body language) can be instantly picked up and exploited by the opposition. Any internal differences within the negotiating team, therefore, need to be identified and brought into the open in advance in order for them to be resolved or accommodated at the preparation stage.

Where more than one person is involved in a side of the negotiation, roles should be allocated. In more formal negotiations, it has been said that 'trying to present a case, chair the management side, and provide a general framework for joint discussion, is akin to trying to referee a football match when you are captain of one of the sides'. Where a number of players are taking part, three clear roles have been identified in the preparation stage:

1. The management of the process.
2. The presentation of the substantive case.
3. The recording of what has been said or agreed.

Roles need to identify and build on team strengths and the advantage of a negotiation involving more than one person on each side is that individual strengths can be exploited to the best advantage and individual weaknesses minimized. However, the preparatory stage is essential in honestly identifying team roles which play to strengths, not weaknesses. It is important to remember that a non-participant with an attention to detail and an ability to observe is as vital as the player who leads the negotiations who, by virtue of their lead role, will inevitably miss the more subtle elements of the negotiation. It is usually the one in the observer/summarizer role who will suggest an adjournment to consider the current state of play and future tactics, and who will point out facts which have gone unnoticed by others in the heat of negotiations.

Opening phase

This is when you exchange as much information as possible and test assumptions made about your opponent's priorities. Make clear any areas you are unable or unwilling to negotiate on. As a guiding principle, your opening should be high if you are 'selling', low if you are 'buying'.

Bargaining phase This is the trading process where concessions should be traded reluctantly and not liberally. It is at this stage that a united front is essential, but where divisions appear if you have not prepared adequately with your negotiating partner(s). Use questioning, not just presenting positions, e.g. 'if I were to give you X, what could you do for me on Y?' Use silence constructively. The inexperienced negotiator finds a silence in this situation uncomfortable and rushes in to fill it, often making further concessions than intended.

Use adjournments – just a brief 'comfort' break to allow you to think about a new direction or proposal, or to do a quick rethink with your negotiating partner. If your partner starts to take a line unplanned, suggest an immediate brief break, without letting your body language display signs of concern. This is a normal 'rule of the game', at worst, your opponent will think you have a weak bladder, at best you will have saved the day!

Make regular summaries of where the negotiations have reached. This helps to keep things on course and clarifies the mind. Now is the time to be soft on people but hard on issues, and separate the people from the problem, where applicable. This is also the time to recognize signals, e.g. listening to what people mean, not just what they say, and to draw on your knowledge of interpersonal skills to identify what underlies other people's behaviour. Your active listening skills are essential at this stage. Similarly, do not let your own body language or tone of voice belie the message you are delivering.

Reaching agreement phase This is when you should achieve a win–win situation using low-cost, high-value solutions. Summarize and make a mutually agreed note of the agreement. Where appropriate, agree on implementation plan, e.g. timescales, individual responsibilities.

STYLE AND STRATEGIES It has become clear that a guiding principle for negotiation strategy can be summarized as shown in Box 5.7.

Box 5.7
Principled negotiations

- ◆ People: separate the people from the problem.
- ◆ Interests: focus on interests, not positions.
- ◆ Options: generate a variety of possibilities before deciding what to do.

The 'people' point highlights the fact that we all have strong emotions, very different perceptions and often do not communicate clearly. Subjective feeling becomes intertwined with the objective issues of the negotiation. People's egos become entangled with their positions. Ideally, participants should see themselves as tackling the problem, not each other.

The 'interests' point will help overcome the problem of focusing on people's stated positions, when it is really their underlying interests which need to be satisfied. Compromising between positions may not produce an agreement which will satisfy real interests.

The 'options' point helps address the problem of coming up with solutions while under pressure. Trying to find a single right solution can inhibit flexibility and creativity. Instead, set aside time to consider a range of possible options that progress shared interests and thus assist in overcoming differences.

An example of principled negotiations, i.e. focusing on people, interests and options, is establishing an out-of-hours service or GP cooperative. Such a negotiation is complex and multilayered, involving:

♦ Achieving agreement within the practice to the principle and how it might operate.
♦ Achieving agreement with neighbouring practices about the principle and operational details.
♦ Achieving agreement with the health authority for funding and support.
♦ Achieving agreement with the LMC (Local Medical Committee), the ambulance service, the landlord of premises, etc.

Failure to take account of the three key factors described will result in concentrating on winning factional battles rather than winning the war. Factional battles can always be resolved through concentrating negotiations on the formula given, and overriding consideration can then be concentrated on winning the war or overall objectives. This illustrates the vital point of team playing in negotiation, which can help prevent one party from becoming locked into a particular aspect of negotiation, which can distort the whole process.

Box 5.8 shows how principled negotiating techniques can replace the more traditional positional bargaining.

Developing a best alternative to a negotiated agreement instead of a bottom line

You negotiated in order to obtain an advantage. If you cannot obtain sufficient advantage, you should know your BATNA because this tactic will prevent you from accepting adversely disadvantageous terms and from rejecting terms which deserve close attention. In contrast, a 'bottom line' set in advance of negotiations can become a tablet of stone which rules out more flexible and creative solutions. It can stop you from making a bad agreement but can also diminish your bargaining power because relative power hinges on how attractive to each party is the option of not reaching agreement.

Box 5.8
The advantages of
principled negotiating
techniques over
traditional positional
bargaining

Problem		Solution
Positional bargaining: the two traditional positions		Change the game: negotiate on the merits

Soft	Hard	Principled
Participants are friends	Participants are adversaries	Participants are problem-solvers
The goal is agreement	The goal is victory	The goal is a wise outcome reached efficiently and amicably
Make concessions to cultivate the relationship	Demand concessions as a condition of the relationship	Separate the people from the problem
Be soft on the people and the problem	Be hard on the problem and the people	Be soft on the people, hard on the problem
Trust others	Distrust others	Proceed independent of trust
Change your position easily	Dig in to your position	Focus on interests, not positions
Make offers	Make threats	Explore interests
Disclose your bottom line	Mislead as to your bottom line	Avoid having a bottom line
Accept one-sided losses to reach agreement	Demand one-sided gains as the price of agreement	Invent options for mutual gain
Search for the single answer: the one *they* will accept	Search for the single answer: the one *you* will accept	Develop multiple options to choose from; decide later
Insist on agreement	Insist on your position	Insist on using objective criteria
Try to avoid a contest of will	Try to win a contest of will	Try to reach a result based on standards independent of will
Yield to pressure	Apply pressure	Reason and be open to reasons; yield to principle, not pressure

Prior examination of what you will do if you do not conclude an agreement can greatly increase your advantage. It will assist your ease in the process, and this will become clear to your opponents, in turn putting them under pressure as it becomes apparent that you are not placing yourself under the constraint of *having* to conclude an agreement.

An example of this might be a negotiation with social services to obtain a link worker who will liaise on behalf of patients with social services and other agencies to obtain services and support for patients in the practice. In this or similar situations involving social services, ground work could usefully be done with the local politicians who control the social services' agenda. Such an approach might be direct or through the HA or relevant agency. However, not *having* to reach a negotiated agreement is a positive advantage. Knowledge of this position may make the social services bureaucracy more receptive to discussions about options for cooperation in an open climate.

Whether to disclose your BATNA up front to the other party depends on how potentially attractive it is. For example, if you are intending to purchase a computer system on the best possible terms, it will strengthen your position if the sales representative knows that you are under no pressure to conclude a deal because your next appointment is with one of his or her competitors. If, on the other hand, this is not the case and your best alternative to a negotiated agreement is worse than your opponent knows, your BATNA should not be disclosed.

A BATNA can also help you in negotiations with another party who is more powerful or influential. The greater your capacity to walk away from a negotiation, the greater your ability to achieve a win–win outcome. This is your greatest protection in dealing with a more powerful negotiator.

***How to counter
underhand tactics***
You know that in reality not everyone will play the same principled game as you. These very principles and your understanding of interpersonal skills is your defence. The golden rule is to understand what the other parties' tactics are, why they are using them and not to fall into the traps they are trying to set up. Dubious tactics will often consist of the other parties aggressively asserting their superior position, and attacking you or your ideas on a personal level. In this situation, practise the principles that have been explained. Do not respond by challenging them or their allegedly superior position. Look for the interests underlying their position and concentrate on these, turn an attack on you into an attack on the problem, and do not indulge in defensive behaviour. Use the weapon of silence, which will not be expected and will usually throw your opponent.

Where tactics adopted are clearly underhand, recognize this immediately and negotiate the rules of the game. Make it plain that you will not discuss substance until you have agreement on procedure. Most people will go along with an uncomfortable situation, hoping to change the rules or gain advantage as they proceed. An experienced negotiator will always clarify the process to be adopted which, in itself, will moderate the other party's behaviour by letting them know that they have been 'found out' and their tactics are not as clever as they had thought! If it is clear that a personal attack is not going to cloud your judgement or put you into a defensive position, such a tactic will usually cease.

Exactly the same rules apply as previously explored. Separate the people from the problem, focus on interests, not positions, think of options for mutual gain and have your BATNA ready.

CONCLUSION Effective negotiation skills are a key factor in ensuring the success of a primary care-led NHS. Contracting for health care in the managed market requires more than the instinctive skills and experience already possessed by many GPs. The best negotiators are aware of the repertoire of techniques and make a habit of practising them and evaluating outcomes, to further refine the art. The private health care sector is more attuned to this market-driven way of doing business, but that does not mean that the private sector is necessarily better at it, simply that it is the normal business ethic. GPs' primary concern is satisfactory access and outcomes of treatment for their patients. Unfortunately, the reality of present-day economics means that clinicians in general practice have to be business managers as much as clinicians in order to obtain the best outcome for patients. This means rethinking the traditional role of GPs, reallocating traditional duties and taking a new look at funds and resources available to undertake this complicated juggling act.

Nurse practitioners and professional managers are likely to become more prominent in the delivery of primary health care, but this should be viewed as an opportunity, not a threat. A guru of general practice, John Fry used to refer to the condition of 'mural dyslexia', i.e. not being able to see the writing on the wall. The lesson of this is to act to take advantage of developing situations – do not just react.

Applying the techniques and lessons in this chapter should be not just useful and essential, but should also be enjoyable. Obtaining what you want out of life, in both home and work environments, is enormously satisfying, particularly when the hurdles seem difficult to overcome. Indeed, practising the negotiating strategies described proves to be a great stress reliever, quite apart from the business advantages gained.

Success breeds success, just as failure leads to failure. Knowing the techniques of achieving a successful outcome and building on each success, leads not only to personal and professional advantages, but to the practitioner becoming a natural and distinctive negotiator.

SUMMARY

This chapter has demonstrated that it is vitally important to GPs to adopt a new approach to the traditional way of conducting negotiations.

Negotiating skills are not inherent, but are learned and the best negotiators practise these to obtain a personal business advantage.

The clear advantages of negotiation skills are in the areas of: personal effectiveness, business advantage, persuasion, conflict-resolution, self-confidence and better communication.

A constructive negotiation enables one to avoid the common pitfalls which start off looking for compromises or how to make the other party back down through 'point-scoring'. Instead, the techniques described enable one to discuss not one's own individual positions on an issue but one's separate interests. From there, matters of common interest can be identified and a mutually satisfactory outcome explored. This achieves a 'win–win' situation. Other approaches often result in 'win–lose' (one party wins but the other party loses, making an ongoing relationship unsatisfactory) or in 'lose–lose' where neither party achieves satisfactory gains. A satisfactory outcome is achieved through equal concentration on the interpersonal skills required, and the conventions and procedures necessary for a successful outcome.

Finally, the Harvard model is explored (now adopted by ACAS), essentially involving being hard on the issues but soft on people, and learning from the lessons of 'principled negotiation'.

FURTHER READING

♦ Fisher, R. and Ury, W. (1983), *Getting to Yes*. Penguin, Harmondsworth.

The *Washington Post* describes this as: "A joy to read for those who delight in concise, lucid, logical exposition." It offers a straightforward, step-by-step, proven method for negotiating personal and professional disputes with getting taken – and without getting nasty!

♦ Kennedy, G., Benson, J and MacMillan, J. (1987), *Managing Negotiations*. Hutchinson, London.

The author runs 'negotiating clinics' and seminars on four continents and is widely published in this area. The book is practical, well written and user friendly.

REFERENCES

Armstrong, M. *How to be an Even Better Manager*. Kogan Page, London.

Fisher, R. and Ury, W. (1983), *Getting to Yes*. Penguin, Harmondsworth.

Kennedy, G. (1987), *Negotiate Anywhere*! Arrow Books Ltd.

Kennedy, G., Benson, J and MacMillan, J. (1987), *Managing Negotiations*. Hutchinson, London.

Porter, C. (1986), *The Negotiating Process*. University of Westminster, Occasional Paper.

Weightman, J. (1993), *Managing Human Resources*. The Institute of Personnel and Development.

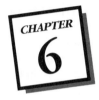

Management of Teams

Ivan Lester and Paul Chapman

OBJECTIVES

- ◆ To examine evolving models of the team approach to management in primary care, together with the problems and challenges facing such an approach.

- ◆ To identify barriers to team work, such as issues of power and control, delegation, empowerment and communication.

- ◆ To explore methods of effective teambuilding and team-working and how to sustain momentum.

- ◆ To examine the future of primary health care teams and the benefits to patients and providers of a multidisciplinary approach.

- ◆ To review examples of current practice, illustrating the above points.

INTRODUCTION

This chapter is intended to promote understanding of the move towards teamwork in primary care. It will illustrate some of the processes involved in the delivery of care by teams and will explore the roles of primary health care teams (PHCTs) in diverse future primary care settings.

Recent legislation has created ample scope for a handful of pioneers to begin innovations that will ripple outwards and alter primary care as drastically as it did in 1948. In particular, once new primary care organizations appear – perhaps involving NHS Trusts, local Social Services Departments and voluntary organizations – a mighty momentum for wide-scale change will grip the system.

Throughout the recent legislation, there are examples of its focus on team delivery of primary care. For example, it is intended that health commissioners will award family health service contracts to 'provider organizations', i.e. PHCTs rather than to general practices and in future 'cost rent' schemes will be geared to buildings housing PHCTs rather than general practitioners (GPs). Following the legislation, the development of PHCTs and interprofessional collaboration will be imperatives.

GPs need more than ever to make themselves aware not only of the benefits of (and barriers to) genuine teamwork in primary care but to acquire the ability to develop and facilitate teamwork in their practices whilst having in mind the diverse models of primary care delivery which are already evolving.

The emerging models exemplified in this chapter require a sound grasp of team management, team organization, team design, team development and the integration of PHCTs into general practice primary care strategies. A proper grasp of the benefits and problems of interprofessional teamworking has become essential basic knowledge for today's general practitioner.

GPs should now be asking themselves:

♦ How and by whom will primary care be provided in the future?
♦ Is there to be an end to the exclusive monopoly of general practice?
♦ Will salaried GPs become the norm?
♦ What kind of new primary care organizations will develop?

This chapter examines the issues surrounding PHCT development and provides a glimpse into the future of a general practice in which teamworking will be an essential ingredient.

Tim Porter O'Grady (1995) identified that the professions have entrenched themselves into separate hierarchical 'silos' in which knowledge is shared vertically with professional peers, but not horizontally amongst other disciplines. He proposed that hierarchies be replaced by professionals coming together as equals to decide the priorities and strategies of health care. This system, called 'shared governance', depends on those involved in the delivery of health care recognizing mutually the importance of the part played by each individual – as in PHCTs.

PHCTs involving GPs and other professionals are already developing throughout the UK. Professionals included are community and primary care nurses, social workers, psychiatric nurses, clinical psychologists, counsellors, dieticians, health visitors, occupational therapists, physiotherapists and pharmacists. This is not an exhaustive list.

In fact, primary care has the advantage of not having to suffer the layers of management which have been increasingly built into secondary care provision during the last 20 years or so. A culture of 'getting ideas out of the heads of bosses and into the heads of labour' (Matsushita, 1995) is less traditional in the primary care setting. There is, however, a tradition of care being delivered to patients by one individual. That is the doctor, sometimes 'assisted' by other professionals. In the rest of the National Health Service (NHS), staff increasingly work around a common purpose rather than in separate compartments.

Because PHCTs now work across the primary/secondary care boundaries and indeed across the boundaries of other agencies, such as local government, catalysing and coordinating service provision to patients becomes of equal importance to the actual supply of service.

The idea of teamwork is not new. In the 1950s the Tavistock Institute, working particularly in the coal mining industry, showed that when groups of miners were organized into teams, given responsibility for a complete part of a process and allowed to set their own performance targets, they were more strongly motivated and achieved higher output than equivalent groups who were set specific tasks and targets on a piecework reward basis.

Before 1948, GPs usually worked single-handedly. During the period 1948–1966 the formation of the Royal College of General Practitioners encouraged a team approach in primary care.

The 1966 Family Doctors' Charter enabled employment of practice staff and 70% of the costs were reimbursed. Thus the role of practice nurses expanded and their number increased. Later practice managers were employed to help with management and administration and an increasing number of other health care professionals have since become involved in primary care.

From 1990 onwards the workload created by the new GP contract increased the need to employ practice nurses and practice managers with proven managerial skills.

Box 6.1
Factors influencing PHCT development

1. Government policies.
2. Patient expectations.
3. The need to maximize efficiency and efficacy in the delivery of health care.
4. The changing nature of work.
5. Barriers and benefits.
6. The management of teams.

IMPORTANT FACTORS IN PHCT WORKING

These are summarized in Box 6.1.

GOVERNMENT POLICIES

The policies of the Department of Health are reflected in the regularly issued Executive Letters (ELs).

EL(94)79 contained the sentence 'team work should embrace both primary and secondary activities with emphasis on clinical team development'. This statement will give considerable support to the formation of PHCTs.

A multidisciplinary approach to the development of health care education is strongly supported by the National Health Service Executive (NHSE). Ken Jarrold, then Human Resource Director of the NHS, in EL(95)96, relating to the recently introduced system for the purchase of education and training for health care professionals, wrote

> ... those commissioning education and training are required to purchase multidisciplinary education and training to help promote multidisciplinary team working in the future.

One of the priorities of this EL is to promote multidisciplinary practice and the cooperation and collaboration of health care professionals,

> ... education commissioners should seek to influence education providers to develop programmes which provide opportunities for shared learning. Education commissioners will need to consider which areas of service provision benefit from multidisciplinary approaches. ... This may well be a priority in primary care community settings. This priority does not imply a threat to existing professional qualifications or to independent professional self regulation. Rather it seeks to stimulate the development of shared learning where this will benefit subsequent professional practice.

In the Health of the Nation document (1992) multiprofessional 'healthy alliances' were referred to as an important way of developing strategies for health promotion and education. The Cumberledge Report (1986) on Community Nursing and the Tomlinson Report (1986) on the future of the London Health Services referred to PHCTs as the preferred way forward.

The move to a primary care-led NHS is giving an enormous stimulus to the development of PHCTs. Teamwork in primary care has been encouraged by the need for community care plans, the coordination of hospital discharge policies, joint purchasing arrangements between health authorities and general practice, and the need to work closely with services provided by local authorities.

The Care in Community Programme has brought much extra work for general practice and GPs, as has the advent of day-case surgery and the increasing tendency for many conditions to be managed by GPs rather than by their hospital counterparts. The management of asthma, diabetes and hypertension are areas in which care is shifting from hospitals to primary care and particularly to PHCTs.

Open access to pathology, physiotherapy and other services has encouraged a retention of patients for treatment in GPs' surgeries. Increasingly, these patients are also being cared for by PHCTs.

The push towards GP consortia is helping to free up funds and the freedoms allow GPs to organize practices in a different way and to employ other health care and care professionals.

PATIENT EXPECTATIONS   Patient involvement in making the decisions about health care commissioning and decisions being made about their own treatment is now an NHSE priority. If patients are to be treated by a team, then patients need to understand that there are benefits in being treated by a team. These benefits need careful explanation. Such detailed information that is necessary should be given at every opportunity and should be referred to in practice literature. The development of end user involvement and patient partnership are now key issues.

THE NEED TO MAXIMIZE HEALTH CARE EFFICIENCY AND EFFICACY   An important issue in primary care is the level of financial resource available. This is limited and will continue to be so for the foreseeable future. It may be that the provision of care by PHCTs is more cost effective than the delivery of care by GPs alone but, so far, there is little evidence of this.

With ever increasing demand upon finite resources, the multiplicity of professional backgrounds involved in the delivery of care by PHCTs can in fact ensure that patients receive the most effective treatment delivered in an efficient way. Sharing the workload with other professionals in areas such as family planning, cervical cytology, health checks for the elderly and the management of some chronic diseases could obviate the need for a practice to recruit an additional GP partner, thus making optimum use of available resources.

THE CHANGING NATURE OF WORK   In the past, society was built upon division of labour. Managers had responsibility and workers carried out the tasks. Now, those doing the work increasingly carry responsibilities and are involved in the decision-making process.

The fact that the way in which work is organized is changing throughout the industrial world must profoundly influence the way in which health care delivery is organized. Thus far, this has perhaps had a greater influence in the delivery of care in hospitals rather than in primary care.

The idea of sharing tasks and responsibilities can be confusing. Belbin (1996a), a leading expert in teamwork, has sought to clarify which work is prescriptive to those with particular skills and which work can be shared. This will be explored in more detail later in the chapter. Team empowerment has widened social responsibility at work but, unless it is carefully handled, it can undermine individual responsibility.

To use teams to maximize patient benefit and to optimize resources implies understanding some of the unique features of teams and team construction. Box 6.2 shows characteristics of teams as opposed to groups, thus demonstrating a clear difference between teamwork and group work.

Box 6.2
Distinctive characteristics of a team

	Team	Group
Size	Limited	Medium or large
Selection	Crucial	Immaterial
Leadership	Shared or rotating	Solo
Perception	Mutual knowledge Understanding	Focus on leader
Style	Role spread Coordination	Convergence Conformism
Spirit	Dynamic interaction	Togetherness Persecution of opponents

Source: Belbin, R.M. (1996b), *Harrogate Public Sector Management Centre Conference Series*, May 1996.

PHCT BENEFITS AND BARRIERS (Devlin, 1996)

Benefits to patients

PCHTs:

♦ Give the right care at the right time by the right person.
♦ Prevent duplication of effort. There is less 'shunting' between agencies.
♦ Minimize 'gaps' in patient care.
♦ Allow crises to be recognized and dealt with more efficiently.
♦ Ensure that patients feel included, more in control of their condition, that they benefit from best practice and understand their treatments better.
♦ Provide care more readily across professional and organizational boundaries.
♦ Raise the standards of care through shared experience.
♦ Improve performance in care when provided by teams sharing common values.
♦ Lead to a reduction in conflicting advice.

Benefits to healthcare professionals

PCHTs:

♦ Help in the recognition and respect of colleagues.
♦ Improve the ability to use skills to best effect.
♦ Facilitate learning.
♦ Aid professional development.
♦ Lead to a more satisfying work environment for those involved.
♦ Help extend traditional roles.
♦ Provide a means of sharing success.
♦ Reduce professional misunderstandings.
♦ Are more flexible, and enhance understanding and response to changing circumstances.

Benefits to NHS/ government

PCHTs:

♦ Can improve effective use of cash from local budgets.
♦ Provide better patient outcomes.

♦ Promote community-based care in line with government strategy.
♦ Help ensure that the total of all skills will be greater than the sum of individual parts.
♦ Make for more effective delivery of care with better outcomes.
♦ Lead to more efficient use of staff allowing specialist skills to be used more effectively.
♦ Promote the need for strategic planning and clear objectives.

Barriers   ♦ Team administration takes time.
♦ Team development and training need time and organization.
♦ Accountability – to whom should the team be accountable. Practice owners, i.e. GPs are often unwilling to share the decision-making process. The assumption that GPs would always be team leaders and that some members of the team will be employees of the GPs, who are also in the team, leads to hierarchical structures. Many GPs are simply interested in delegating work and shifting workload, not in shifting accountability and responsibility.
♦ The need to manage across local authority and NHS boundaries, and across primary and secondary care boundaries in the NHS. Health and social services have different management structures and legal frameworks. GPs are usually self-employed, independent contractors. Other health care professionals may be employed by a local NHS Trust, or even by a local authority, leading to difficulties of cross-functional management and difficulties with cross-functional budgeting.
♦ Lack of recognized audit procedures.
♦ GPs are not skilled in resource management or in team management.
♦ Communication barriers.
♦ Lack of clarity of roles within teams.
♦ Different training backgrounds and thus different cultural values between different professional groups.
♦ The inequity of status and pay between team members.
♦ Teams may have the required mix of professional roles but not of 'teambuilding' roles (see Figure 6.1).

Despite these barriers, there have been many examples of excellent and progressive contribution to health care delivery by PHCTs and currently there are a number of experiments involving local authority staff and PHCTs working together.

THE MANAGEMENT OF TEAMS

We are going to win and the industrial West is going to lose. There is nothing much you can do about it, because the reasons for your failure are within yourselves. With your bosses doing the thinking while the workers wield the screwdrivers, you are convinced this is the right way to run a business. For you the essence of management is getting the ideas out of the heads of the bosses and into the hands of labour. (Matsushita, 1995)

PHCTs are about the profound cultural change from a hierarchical approach with all responsibility for care in the hands of one professional – the doctor – to a team approach, where responsibility and accountability for the provision of patient care and treatment is afforded to a team of professionals of equal status, but different professional inputs.

Professor Tony Butterworth of Manchester University believes:

It is necessary to gently destabilise the status quo and gently deconstruct that which already exists in order to develop a more effective organisation.

Teams do not mean *no* individual responsibility. In some matters there must be individual responsibility and in others team responsibility. Primary care development needs to be within a strategic management framework.

The challenge is:

to pierce the fog of uncertainty and develop great foresight. It is a view of strategy that recognises the need for more than an incrementalist, annual planning rain dance; what is needed is a strategic architecture that provides a blueprint for building the competencies needed tomorrow. (Hamel and Prahalad, 1994)

General practice needs to seek out the most effective and efficient model for managing patient care. It needs to forecast strategically what the best model is likely to be, say, 5 years hence because the pathway to that model will decide what is to be done today and tomorrow.

If practices themselves do not have a clear strategy, it will be very difficult for PHCTs to have clear goals. Team goals need to be directly linked to the achievement of an overall strategic plan and regular appraisal of team activity should take into account practice medium- and long-term strategic objectives. PHCTs must be encouraged to evolve within the framework of strategic plans.

Organizational design of teams

Teams are most effective when the totality of the organization is designed around interlocking teams, each with its own purpose, but with each of those purposes linked to the goals and directions of the whole practice. Ideally, these teams will be organized around core processes rather than specialist functions to ensure the activities and tasks of the team are defined by patient requirements, and not individual function or internal goals.

It is possible for individual teams to be successful, including those which must cross over functional boundaries, provided that:

♦ The existence and purpose of the team is accepted by the organization as a whole, for example, a team set up for a specific project or with clear time boundaries is easily recognized and usually regarded as helpful.

♦ The inputs needed by the team are readily available, including finance and information (this often means crossing the traditional 'need to know' boundaries of information availability and has a special relevance with regard to access to patients' medical records).

♦ The outputs of the team are delivered in such a way that the rest of the organization's skill structures in traditional functions and departments can use them effectively within the limits of their own authority/capability. Outputs which require the whole practice organization to be redesigned to make the most of them will probably damage the team's effectiveness and even continued existence. It is often the case that the formation of 'teams for purpose', such as project teams, is the first step towards the organization as a whole understanding the value of teams. Successful project teams can lead to a wider organizational change.

Status   Where status exists – in the sense that some individuals are treated, or are perceived to be treated, as having more value to the organization than others – then teamwork inevitably fails. The complexity of modern organizations requires different skills and competencies and these skills and competencies will attract differential rewards based on the market (scarcity/supply/demand). That is, of course, the situation in the private sector, but with the creation of a market in health care in the NHS, this is beginning to have an effect in the public sector.

Each role requires different skills and competencies. It is important to gain the organization's agreement that within the team there will be equality of status, all contributions equally valued and all team members will share in the risks and rewards of the team's achievement of purpose, even if those rewards are intangible. In the NHS it is clearly not yet possible to change the historic approach to reward based on professional grading, time served and status, and indeed these may have less influence on status in a primary care context.

Rewards and benefits   There are some examples of team rewards and benefits in the secondary health care sector, but few at the present time in the context of PHCTs. Most reward and benefit systems underpin the organizational hierarchy and do not acknowledge, motivate or reward individual development, nor individual and team contribution. They also do not recognize individual circumstances or requirements. There is a desire for uniformity. This is true of nationally agreed pay rates in the NHS. This will not change overnight, it will evolve as changing work and life patterns force change. It is important, however, that for a team to be successfully motivated:

♦ There must be some element of reward or recognition of team achievement. The criteria for reward for achievement must be the same for all team members (but not necessarily the amount of such reward).

♦ The team should have an input into how the reward is distributed amongst team members based on their assessment of their performance. It is easier to change or supplement reward systems in GP fundholding practices, but only for those team members employed directly by the practices. In most organizations, performance appraisal is based on the manager–subordinate relationship, even though managers may have little knowledge or experience of how these individuals perform their tasks on a day-to-day basis and particularly do not know how they relate to other individuals in the organization. Teams will see and experience first hand how team colleagues behave and perform. They, therefore, should have an input into the appraisal of other team members, even if it is through the team leader.

Management process/audit   It is often difficult to fit the management of teams into traditional methods of management and, in many organizations, the process of management has arisen *ad hoc* and is not strategically developed. Most management reviews divide the evaluation of an organization's performance into discrete activities, such as finance, operations, resources, etc., whereas it is the essence of team management to evaluate the performance of a team as a whole against agreed objectives/purpose. The 'management process' thus needs to be adapted to ensure that the team's performance can be measured holistically against agreed requirements. Without large-scale research, the ultimate effectiveness of teamworking in relation to patients is difficult to measure.

Consider the workings of an asthma clinic. How is it possible to assess whether or not the team is doing a good job in improving patients' health without substantial resources devoted to research? Whilst it is difficult to assess an improvement in morbidity, it is certainly possible to audit the way in which the team is working and to audit processes. So, for example, questions which could be asked and easily answered include:

♦ What percentage of asthmatic patients attend clinics?
♦ Were agreed protocols for treatment followed?
♦ What was the degree of patient satisfaction?
♦ Did the organization of the clinic affect other activities in the practice?

These and other questions could be used as a basis for audit.

Every so often teams need to break from their routine consideration and tasks to take time to review their own effectiveness. As they set their own norms and performance measures, they are the only ones who can assess the effectiveness. It sometimes makes such sessions more fruitful if they are conducted away from a work environment. There are many methods that can be used. One simple approach consists of three questions.

♦ What has been done well and what can be improved.
♦ What has been done well from which all can learn.
♦ Are there any other issues, ideas or opportunities, or concerns.

Management style The more traditional style of management in many organizations, often called 'command and control' style, does not sit well with teams. In fact, many managers who have risen in organizations by demonstrating that they are tough on setting objectives, hard on less than effective performance and are experts in their particular function or speciality, find the whole concept of teams threatening. This certainly applies to some health care professionals. It is the teams who are the experts, not the manager or the individual professional. What they require from their 'team manager' is constant support for their aims and resource requirements in the management process, protecting the team against adverse influences, and coaching and counselling from wider experience. Sympathetic and even empathetic management is needed to nurture teams, particularly at the beginning. In an interprofessional team, the management role could be simply that of a facilitator bringing out the best of a group of professionals from different backgrounds, who are working together.

Team direction It is almost impossible to implement effective teams in any organization without the support of either the whole of the 'direction team', e.g. the GP partners or as a minimum a powerful sponsor, e.g. a practice senior partner, who is prepared to take necessary action to facilitate the team success. If those ultimately responsible for success do not see teams as adding enhanced performance, then it is unlikely that, however committed the team members are to their values, purpose and each other, they will succeed.

Team design The need to manage services through PHCTs requires different practices and skills from those which are required in secondary care. It is important that staff be allowed to negotiate the way they work rather than being rigidly confined to traditional systems.

Case studies In these three examples, a Trust has worked with the GPs on evaluation and protocols. Now, other GPs, fundholding and non-fundholding practices in Leeds are interested to 'buy' into the scheme using their own funds.

Case study 1

> The Leeds Mental Health and Community NHS Trust has helped in a pilot project to develop three PHCTs each of which is different.
>
> In a seven-doctor GP fundholding practice, a PHCT has been formed in which the team leader is a health visitor (and is given extra pay to work as team leader). The 'team brief' comes from the practice manager and the 'direction' from the general practitioners. Technical, secretarial and functional support is provided by the Trust, which stays at arms length from the team, but helped initially and helps set performance indicators. The PHCT is practice based and works entirely on its own core services but receives support services from the Trust. The Trust is still the employer of its own staff and is responsible for their education, training and development. The Trust exercises no authority – that lies with the practice manager. Members of the team have found this work to be 'a very enjoyable experience sharing common values'. Anecdotal evidence is that patients are not in fact aware that they are being treated by a PHCT as opposed to a GP. A common caucus of senior partners attend team meetings, other GPs attend occasionally.

Case study 2

> In another Leeds practice, there is a large multidisciplinary team which includes a community midwife who unusually is paid and seconded by a local acute Trust. The workings of this team could be described as 'two cog wheels moving together and then moving apart – they interface but are not joined and they mesh when necessary'. The exclusivity of medical practice is maintained but a place is created for other professionals. There is close cooperation between health care professionals, and individual members of the team occasionally negotiate their own methods of working. Prior to the development of team working, a community midwife would hand over childcare to a health visitor 2 days post partum. This has been changed to a handover at 14 days and the care in the first 14 days is shared between a midwife and a health visitor

often on a geographical basis with each attending to different clients. The Leeds Mental Health and Community NHS Trust has involvement at arms length and the matter of who actually pays the staff appears to be immaterial, but the fact that there is a Community Trust in the background solves the problem of professional 'back up' and professional education and training.

A system of appraisal called performance management review has been introduced and financial activity, 'client' relations, innovation and change, and strategic outlook are reviewed. The review is carried out by Leeds Community Healthcare Trust managers, even for those not employed by the Trust. Management is by 'a quiet word spoken across professional lines without formality'.

Case study 3

In a third example, the staff attached to the Community Trust work as a team but, in this case, the Community Trust puts more time into managing that team and the Trust managers work closely with the practice manager to organize the work. It is admitted that there is some confusion about 'who is in charge'. The process in this case needs a higher level of skill in working together than the other two and management is more hierarchical.

The Community Trust, although paying for some practice staff, feels that it is benefiting because, with other general practices in the city being interested, the Trust's income stream is likely to increase – and will also increase because other Trust services are being increasingly purchased, e.g. rehabilitation services and the provision of primary care psychiatric nurses and mobile rehabilitation consultant sessions at GP premises.

It is clear that the Community Trust, the GP practices and the patients all benefit from these arrangements.

The nature of different teams for different purposes

Team of teams

In this situation the whole organization is a set of interlocking teams. The members of the teams will be permanent (until moved to another 'permanent' team), but also the leaders of each team will be members of another permanent team along with their fellow team leaders. A useful example is a social services team working alongside a PHCT. These teams will each be led by managers who themselves could be members of a management team, led by a director who is then part of the direction management team. Each team has a purpose and a set of rules and responsibilities, and the interlocking membership ensures that the sum of the achievement of all these purposes will fulfil the direction of the organization as in the second Leeds example.

Teams for purpose

Some organizations frequently use teams to achieve a specific purpose. Project teams are probably the best example of this. This enables an organization to deliver cross-functional change programmes, whilst keeping a traditional structure in place. So a project team might be set up in a primary care context to input into a health authority's strategic plans for commissioning health care in the district. Quite often the contrast in working styles between the team and the more traditional functions or departments, and the personal development absorbed by individuals who have worked in a team, lead to radical organizational change based on teams. Project teams tend to do their work together, at meetings and to disband when the project is completed.

Virtual teams

There are certain circumstances where, to fulfil the purpose of the team, the same skills, roles and responsibilities are always required, but it might not be possible to keep the same individuals together. These are known as virtual teams. A typical example would be an operating theatre team in a hospital.

Self-managing teams

It is possible, particularly where teams have worked together for a long time and are very clear about their roles and responsibilities, for there not to be a clearly identified team leader role. Frequently different members of the team will fill the role for a specified period or for a specified purpose (as in the first Leeds example).

Whatever form the team takes, depending on the circumstances and environment, there are a number of key characteristics of behaviour, methods and management which make for an effective team.

Characteristics of successful teams   There are many views about what makes an effective team. There are a number of characteristics which are common to effective teams. These are described below (Box 6.3) in no particular order of importance, as depending on the circumstances, the environment and the culture in which the team exists, different characteristics will assume different priorities (Belbin, 1993).

Team leadership

There is no one particular style which makes someone an effective team leader, in fact, effective team leaders have to adopt many different styles according to circumstances. Leaders need to behave

Box 6.3
Essential
characteristics of an
effective team

♦ Shared purpose and vision – common values.

♦ Good communication between all participants.

♦ Clear and appropriate objectives – protocols for specific clinical procedures.

♦ Regular assessment of progress. Audit.

♦ Mutual trust, honesty, understanding, respect and support.

♦ A leader who is able to coordinate and facilitate.

♦ All the necessary individual specialist skills, but willingness and ability to support others and to fill in gaps.

♦ The need for clear responsibilities for performance management and resource management.

♦ Confidence in confidentiality.

♦ A process for team development and the identification of training needs.

differently in different situations. The strengths and weaknesses of individual members of the team, a changing external environment and different behaviours within the team all have influence. The team leader needs to be trained to recognize these different situations and how to deal with each one effectively, balancing all the time the three key factors of the team, the individual and the task.

A clear purpose

Effective teams have a clear purpose and time should be spent by the team leader in getting the team to understand fully this purpose, the requirement that it creates, the implications for the team, the organization and the individuals. If the team does not fully understand the purpose, cohesion will suffer. A typical purpose for a PHCT would be to provide the best possible care in the most effective, efficient way which will give patient satisfaction, and which will lead to a satisfactory clinical and social response in the patient.

Competencies

A traditional, functional organization tends to rely on the functional specialism and skill of the individual to achieve objectives. In a team, however, individual skills are not enough. What is more important is how the individual is able to apply those skills, both to fulfil their own roles and to help others in the team understand the issues and resolutions. Thus, planning, creativity and project management become key competencies to support the specialist professional or technical skills, and behavioural skills need to be developed.

Team size

Theoretically, it is possible for a team to be any size given a common purpose, including defined roles and responsibilities, but for practical purposes most teams seem to be most effective when the number of members does not exceed about ten.

Team roles and responsibilities

Although one of the key benefits that effective teams bring to an organization is that the total is greater than the sum of the parts, this can only be achieved if every individual has a clear understanding of their own role and responsibilities. The rest of the team will rely on this and will operate in the belief that each fulfil their own responsibilities. As well as their own specific role and responsibilities related to the purpose or task, individuals also have a natural team role. Thus, some individuals are good at assessing and developing ideas and options, less good at implementing them. Others are more natural producers or implementers, and there are individuals who would tend more readily to go outside the team to bring ideas back in. Where these natural roles are well balanced, it improves the effectiveness of the team and the team leader's role needs to be less interventionist. Where the natural roles are not well balanced, team sessions can be difficult. An inherent weakness in human nature is the tendency to judge others by a mirror of oneself, thus it is easy to recruit a team of people reflecting one's own strengths when one should be recruiting to complement those strengths and to support weak areas.

There are a number of different methods of assessing team roles. The Belbin method is probably the best known (Figure 6.1). In order to gain full value of the insight into team effectiveness, it is usually necessary to use a specialist human resource adviser or consultant.

THE IMPORTANCE OF TEAM DEVELOPMENT

Team development in general practice needs to be a part of wider primary care development and should include clinicians, providers, managers and users. A Leeds Family Health Services PHCT development project (personal communication) proved relatively unsuccessful because development and training were focused on individual team members rather than on the team as a whole.

The NHSE's requirement for interdisciplinary education has been outlined earlier. If hospitals are traditionally the venues in which medical and other health care professional education takes place, and there are fewer and fewer hospitals, then health care education

Figure 6.1
Belbin team-role profile

Roles and descriptions (team-role contribution)	Allowable weaknesses
Plant: Creative, imaginative, unorthodox. Solves difficult problems.	Weak in communicating with and managing ordinary people.
Resource investigator: Extrovert, enthusiastic, communicative. Explores opportunities. Develops contacts.	Loses interest once initial enthusiasm has passed.
Coordinator: Mature, confident and trusting. A good chairman. Clarifies goals, promotes decision-making.	Not necessarily the most clever or creative member of a group.
Shaper: Dynamic, outgoing, highly strung. Challenges, pressurizes, finds ways round obstacles.	Prone to provocation and short-lived bursts of temper.
Monitor evaluator: Sober, strategic and discerning. Sees all options. Judges accurately.	Lacks drive and ability to inspire others.
Teamworker: Social, mild, perceptive and accommodating. Listens, builds, averts friction.	Indecisive in crunch situations.
Implementer: Disciplined, reliable, conservative and efficient. Turns ideas into practical actions.	Somewhat inflexible, slow to respond to new possibilities.
Completer: Painstaking, conscientious, anxious. Searches out errors and omissions. Delivers on time.	Inclined to worry unduly. Reluctant to delegate.
Specialist: Single-minded, self-starting, dedicated. Provides knowledge or technical skills in rare supply.	Contributes on only a narrow front.

Source: Belbin, R. M. (1996b), *Harrogate Public Sector Management Centre Conference Series*, May 1996.

will have to take place somewhere else – and will move into primary care context.

Only when health care professionals are educated together, even if that means common core subjects, or a common foundation degree in health care studies, will they truly respect each others abilities in such a way as to allow proper teamwork. In the meantime, time spent on team development and training will bring considerable rewards.

Teams tend to rely heavily on problem-solving tools and methods. That is because the success of a team depends upon making the full use of the potential of the specialist skills of all its members. As these members will have been trained for different functional roles or specialisms, it is important to use general methods which will be universally understood by everyone. A very simple method to structure the resolution of a problem is to ensure that everyone understands the issues in the same way. This method consists of three questions and has become known as the 3Q approach (Figure 6.2).

Figure 6.2
Redesigning an organization: the 3Q approach

RE-DESIGNING AN ORGANIZATION

The Three Questions

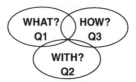

CREATING THE DIRECTION

Q1 What do we want to do:

- Mission
- Goals
- Strategy
- Values
- Philosophy of management
- Agree the statement of the problem or issue so that everybody shares the same understanding

AGREEING THE REQUIREMENTS

Q2 With what do we need to do it:

- Roles and responsibilities
- Management processes
- Management system
- Identification of all the information and inputs needed to address the problems at the beginning of the process

Q3 How are we to do it?

- Implementation processes
- Implementation systems
- Roles and responsibilities
- Criteria for evaluation

Figure 6.3
The team management cycle

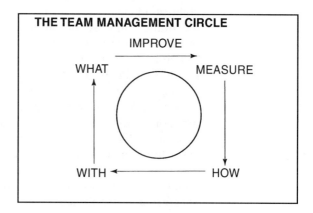

THE TEAM MANAGEMENT CIRCLE

Team meetings
- ◆ Everyone who has a role in the topics to be discussed should be involved.
- ◆ In large practices, representatives of interest groups can be chosen to attend.
- ◆ Task-oriented meetings may provide a good option.
- ◆ Meetings should be held in convenient locations at convenient times.
- ◆ The success of a meeting depends heavily on the quality of chairmanship and facilitation.
- ◆ The length of the agenda is critical.
- ◆ Everyone should have an opportunity to express their views.
- ◆ Tasks allocated at a meeting should be carefully minuted and clear instructions sent after the meeting to the people concerned.

It is helpful in team sessions to appoint a facilitator to write all inputs and outputs on flip charts so that these are always visible to the team. It is also useful that flip charts are copied and circulated. There are many different problem-solving tools available; the simpler these are the better. The important point is that the team should be comfortable with the tools being used.

Team norms
It usually makes sense for a team to agree 'norms' of operation. Simple issues like time to be spent on an issue, who will facilitate, who will write up a report, etc. Whilst these norms might seem almost too simple, failure to agree them in advance and to adhere to them can have a severe detrimental effect on the quality of the considerations and output of the team.

Team resource
This is the factor that usually causes the most contention. Although teams can manage the resource more effectively in an environment which requires nimbleness and flexibility, there is a prerequisite that, having agreed their purpose and roles and responsibilities with the organization, they must be given the necessary resources to achieve that purpose. Clear parameters must be agreed about financial and human resources, and the team must be allowed to allocate resources to its best ability. Teams should not be seen by the organization as a means of reducing resource or the concept of teamwork will lose its value.

EXAMPLES OF EMERGING PRIMARY HEALTH CARE PROVIDER MODELS
1. Local PHCTs are helping develop the health authority's purchasing plans in the Wessex Region (Meads, 1996) and, in Andover, several fundholding practices and the local community hospital are seeking to join forces to produce a new 'primary care agency'. This would become a federation or cooperative of small health care 'businesses' led by GPs and incorporating many community health

services. The model promotes closer working between GP practices and local hospital management. Many of the responsibilities
for primary care and purchasing would be delegated to this
primary care agency. This project also involves greater involvement
of the local community in health affairs. Merging the Trust with the
local GP fundholding practices would involve putting outpatient
services out to tender, thus the Trust would become the purchaser
and provider of services, i.e. a primary care agency constructed
loosely around the US 'health maintenance organization' model.
The agency would be directed by a board of GPs working alongside
business managers.

2. Another model, the City Multi-Fund, is found in Southampton
(Meads, 1996). This is a local association of fundholding GP
practices which came together to form a cooperative group. Some
of the management allowance is pooled collectively to form a
strong purchasing team acting on behalf of the practices. The Multi-
Fund represents some 60% of the local population and sees itself
influencing health care strategies beyond the boundaries currently
covered within the remit of GP fundholding. Being an association
of independent practices, it can develop as a body whilst at the
same time respecting a diversity of approach. It allows GPs to
develop a common training package bringing together GPs and
practice managers, and the fund is able to build a picture of overall
needs of the community and develop a locality healthcare plan. It
also allows GPs to negotiate on an equal footing with powerful local
providers.

3. An interesting model is Patrick Pietroni's Marylebone Health
Centre (Meads, 1996). This is a general practice experimenting
with different models of delivering primary care. The practice
includes a counselling and psychotherapy unit, a social care unit
with outreach workers, a health promotion and health education
unit, complementary therapies and a patient participation programme.

4. The Primary Care Trust (Meads, 1996) is a radical idea, a Trust
which is formed by the merger of provider functions of independent contractor partnerships and the local Community Trust. It
would control most resources for purchasing secondary care
services and be accountable to a health authority for its performance. Ideally, GPs would become members of the Trust and
receive a share of its profits, and others would have a salary
option. Some GP partnerships might seek an affiliated membership. Such a Trust could be in the independent sector and the
independent contractor status could be maintained. The management would largely be in the hands of its members. It would
contract with the health authority for such services as general
medical services, childhealth services, family planning services,
health visiting, primary and community nursing, dietetics, physiotherapy, chiropody and occupational therapy. Other services may

be agreed with the health authority. On the 'ownership board' could be represented the local authority and the local university voluntary groups and others.

5. The Lyme Regis Scheme (Meads, 1996) is influenced by the American system of 'managed care'. The Lyme Community Care Unit was founded in 1992 to provide a solution to the provision of an integrated and social care services to all citizens living in the locality regardless of their address or GP. Its purpose is to translate the complex web of services providers and purchaser into a single organizational model whose care was centred on the citizen whilst it retained the accountability to statutory agencies. It has the status of a limited company and was set up by GPs working in the locality, but is an independent and separate entity. The professionals and areas which are represented within the team employed by the Lyme Community include community nursing, hospital at home, physiotherapy, occupational therapy, social worker, chiropody, casualty, health visiting, dietician, speech therapy, community psychiatric nurse, school nurse, counsellor, GPs, care manager, midwife and community health adviser. There is a management advisory group helping transfer its possibility for health and social well-being from the statutory body to the citizen. One of the GPs acts as part-time unit general manager.

6. A Hereford and Worcester practice has an attached social worker included in their primary health care team. The team includes a community nurse, a school nurse, a health visitor for the elderly, two paediatric health visitors, an occupational therapist, a chiropodist and a locality manager. From time to time a general psychiatrist and a psychiatrist for the elderly hold outpatient clinics. A study showed that the attachment of a qualified social worker to provide care management for disabled people was successful in generating a greater uptake of community care services and financial benefits, and was effective in removing the usual problems of poor liaison. This project was funded by the social services department.

7. The Salford Family Health Services Authority, together with Salford Social Services and Salford Community Health Care Trust, have set up the Salford Pass Project (Meads, 1996) which aims to create a mechanism of greater understanding between general practice and social work. Those involved include GPs, practice staff, and the social care team as well as the community staff, including district nurses, health visitors, midwives and community psychiatric nurses. At meetings, difficulties are explored in terms of specific patients or incidents. Typical problems include not knowing when to make a referral, asking for information that is not forthcoming and not receiving feedback on referrals.

CONCLUSION
- ◆ The NHS (Primary Care) Act (1996) will profoundly affect the future. No health professional is an island insulated from change elsewhere. Trust status and fundholding were voluntary when introduced but have proceeded at a pace which has transformed the NHS within an initial period of time.
- ◆ Diverse models for the delivery of primary care are developing even now without the need for legislative change and 'pilots' are being supported by the NHS Executive. The need to reduce so-called 'transaction costs' will push governments of whatever complexion to promote the reorganization of primary care.
- ◆ Consideration of just a few of the examples of emerging primary care organizations gives a glimpse into likely developments in the future involving new types of organization of care delivery.
- ◆ The independent sector is expressing interest in providing funds for the development of other types of emerging model.
- ◆ Merging primary care and community care is appearing as one future pattern perhaps combining the entrepreneurial skills of GPs alongside the management capability of the Community NHS Trusts.
- ◆ GP fundholding seems likely to be superseded by locality commissioning and other new models. GPs may increasingly become salaried employees being employed directly as members of PHCT.

What is clear is that general practice must seize the initiative, be proactive and take advantage of the political will towards PHCT working. A valuable opportunity to shape and be at the forefront of enhancing primary care must not be lost!

The point of the game is not how well the individual does, but whether the team wins. That is the beautiful part of the game, the blending of personalities, the mutual sacrifices for group success. (Bradley, 1994).

SUMMARY

In the light of proposed new legislation, the delivery of primary health care by teams will increase considerably.

- ◆ The primary health care team as we know it has developed largely in response to political, organizational and clinical pressures.
- ◆ Training is required for team members deficient in necessary team skills.
- ◆ Training development should be directed to whole teams.
- ◆ The personal responsibility of each member within the team framework must be identified and accepted.
- ◆ Patients should encounter the teams, not unconnected co-workers.

- Every member of the practice should participate in quality assurance and audit.
- The result of effective teamwork should be, primarily, an increased quality of care.
- An explanation of the benefit of care by PHCTs must be available to patients.
- Primary care throughout the world is undergoing a revolution. The nature of delivery of care is changing rapidly as is the nature of the care delivered. During the early part of the next century, change will be promoted by major advances in information technology including telemedicine as well as in the scientific basis of medicine.
- PHCTs are beginning to operate in a very different primary care environment to that which applied hitherto. Some elements of primary care are now external to GP practices and this trend will continue. This release of the control of care from GP partnerships will make an enormous difference.
- There are a few examples of other professionals becoming partners in general practices.
- Doctors will increasingly have to accept integration as equals into teams of health care professionals.
- Increasingly the PHCT is extending beyond the boundaries of GP practices.
- The merger of FHSAs into health authorities, with all the resource implications that that brings, has been a powerful catalyst for change.
- Health and social care will become increasingly integrated, emphasizing the need for an interprofessional approach.
- Funds from different sources will be applied – hospital and community trusts, general medical services, local authority social services, charities and health insurers and the private sector.
- The medical profession will continue to provide a service to new organizations and are likely to continue as independent contractors, but they may not be the exclusive stakeholders in the new teams.
- GP skills are clinical and they are not usually managerial. There is arising a profession of 'care management' with an accreditation in which primary health care staff are trained in the management function and then accredited. This will enable them to acquire access to local authority budgets and services, and reduce duplication and decision making by different agencies. In Wiltshire (Meads, 1996), there is a proposal to allocate indicative community budgets to a number of PHCTs and GP fundholders and the social services department are working to develop parallel local purchasing plans. Wiltshire is working with the Kings Fund to review the pattern of services available for elderly people and their carers and jointly commis-

sion between health and social services. It is clear that a more integrated social services and primary health care is on the way.

♦ There are many examples of public and private collaboration in public and primary health care (Meads, 1996). PHCTs are becoming the norm rather than the exception, and taking time to understand how teams work and in developing the management of teams will bring considerable rewards for general practice, for primary care as a whole and for patients.

FURTHER READING

♦ Meads, G. (ed.) (1996), *Future Options for General Practice*. Radcliffe Medical Press, Oxford.

An excellent compendium of new and diverse primary care organizations.

♦ Pringle, M. (1993), *Change and teamwork in primary care*. British Medical Journal, London.

A detailed exposition of team work in relation to expected changes in primary care.

♦ Belbin, R. M. (1996), *The coming shape of organisation*. Butterworth Heinemann, Oxford.

♦ Belbin R. M. (1993), *Team rule at work*. Butterworth Heinemann, Oxford.

♦ Pritchard and Pritchard (1994), *Team work for primary and shared care*. Oxford University Press, Oxford.

REFERENCES

Belbin, R. M. (1993), *Team Role Profile. Team Roles at Work*. Butterworth Heinemann, Oxford.
Belbin, R. M. (1996a), *The Coming Shape of Organisations*. Butterworth Heinemann, Oxford.
Belbin, R. M. (1996b), *Harrogate Public Sector Management Centre Conference Series*, May.
Bradley, B. (1994), *Life on the Run*.
Cumberledge Report on Community Nursing (1986).
Devlin, M. (1996), *Chemist and Druggist* 16 March and 6 April.
Hamel, G. and Prahalad, C. K. (1994), *Competing for the Future*. Harvard Business School Press.
Harrogate Public Sector Management Series (1996), November.
Health of the Nation (1992), Secretary of State.
Matsushita, M. K. (1995), Matsuhita Electric Industrial Corporation.
Meads, G. (ed.) (1996), *Future Options for General Practice*. Radcliffe Medical Press, Oxford.
The NHS (Primary Care) Act 1996.
Porter O'Grady, T. (1995), *Nursing Management* **2**, 6 October.
Tomlinson Report, The Future of the London Health Services (1986).

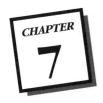

CHAPTER 7

STATUTORY AND LEGAL RESPONSIBILITIES

Peter Hildebrand

OBJECTIVES

- ◆ To increase awareness of legal concepts as they affect all aspects of business and professional relationships.

- ◆ To promote an analytical approach to legal issues facing the practitioner.

- ◆ To prevent action being taken before the legal consequences have been considered.

INTRODUCTION

This chapter aims to provide an outline of certain important aspects in which the legal framework affects doctors in general practice. In particular these are:

- ◆ Relationships with partners and employees in the practice.
- ◆ Relationships with patients.
- ◆ The underlying legal framework comprising the doctor's responsibility to the health authority.
- ◆ The regulators.

There is no area of daily life that is not subject to a significant degree of legal regulation and this is particularly the case in general medical practice. The aim of this chapter is not to provide a definitive answer to the many issues which arise but to set out the areas where the practising physician may encounter regulation and to outline the form that regulation may take.

RELATIONSHIPS WITH PARTNERS AND EMPLOYEES

Partnership – strengths and weaknesses

Partnership is the relation which subsists between persons carrying on a business in common with a view of profit.

Despite the archaic language, this definition taken from the Partnership Act 1890 remains the operative definition in analysing whether a partnership exists. This is an issue which is ultimately decided by a court despite that which the parties involved may

This chapter aims to state the law as at 1st March 1997.

have decided was the legal nature of their relationship. A partnership can be formed by written agreement or it can be created by conduct, and there is no requirement for formality or writing. This can have extremely far reaching effects. The primary statutory source in this context is the Partnership Act 1890. The firm which is created by a partnership does not have any separate identity. The main consequence is that every partner becomes an agent of the firm and his or her other partners for the purposes of carrying on the business. Every partner in a firm is liable jointly with the other partners for all debts and obligations of the firm. It is particularly important to note that a person who is admitted as a partner into an existing firm does not become liable to the creditors of the firm for anything done before he or she became a partner. If follows that a partner who retires from a firm does not thereby cease to be liable for partnership debts or obligations incurred before his or her retirement.

Other important aspects to mention are that no majority of partners can expel a partner unless power to do so has been confirmed by express agreement between the partners. Where no fixed term has been agreed for the duration of the partnership, any partner may bring the partnership to an end at any time on giving notice of his or her intention so to do to all the partners. This is a most unsatisfactory position for a partnership to face and for this reason alone it is desirable that a properly considered partnership agreement should be in force at the earliest opportunity. Even if there was an arrangement for a fixed term which continues after the term has expired, without any express new agreement, the rights and duties of the partners remain as before insofar as this is consistent with a 'partnership at will', in other words a continuation of the partnership as long as the partners agree.

By way of summary, while a partnership can provide an extremely flexible and resilient method of organization, by the same token it can prove to be a haven for the most intractable of disputes if trust disappears between the partners. It should also be made clear that, as a matter of law, the partners owe each other a duty of the 'utmost good faith'. For these reasons, and particularly because of the lack of formality and structure imposed by the general law, it is imperative that any properly constituted partnership should have an agreement dealing with the important issues in the management and interrelations of the partnership. In the absence of agreement, the court will supervise the winding up of a partnership.

The partnership agreement   The key clauses of the partnership agreement are shown in Box 7.1.

The partnership agreement should provide a clear framework for how the partnership is to operate. Important matters that need to be addressed at the outset include the question of capital. The partnership should carefully consider how its capital is treated in

Box 7.1
Key clauses of the
partnership agreement

1. Contributions of capital
2. Holding of assets
3. Share of profits
4. Liability for debts
5. Duties of partners
6. Authority of partners
7. New entrants
8. Leave
9. Medical records
10. Expenses
11. Termination provisions/restrictions

the accounts and the extent to which incoming partners should be obliged to contribute to that capital. It may provide for an initial capital fund to be paid in respect of the partnership equipment and it may also provide for an incoming partner to agree to a restriction in drawings of profit to allow a capital share to accumulate. The agreement should also specify what property, if any, is held by the partners on trust for the partnership as a whole so that it is clear whether, for example, partnership property is being rented from a former partner or held by the continuing partners for the benefit of the partnership. Normally partners who have capital invested in a partnership are entitled to receive interest to reflect the fact that they have invested their capital in the partnership other than elsewhere. Any deficiency on capital account by a partner should be recognized by an obligation to pay interest to the partnership on account of the fact that other partners are investing greater sums of capital to accommodate the deficiency.

The agreement should also make clear the method of division of partnership profits. This is an extremely important area where the strength of the organization can be measured. For it to survive and go forward, any organization must provide a just system of rewards for the participants. In an unduly rigid system, there will be no scope for change when greater seniority is acquired. It may be that partners will want to accept a lesser share of responsibility in return for a reduced share of the profits at a later stage in their careers. Normally, the agreement will stipulate the level of drawing which is allowed on account of profits. The agreement should also deal with arrangements, such as holidays and rota working, and may go into the partners' obligations in terms of time to be devoted to the partnership. The agreement will also set out the terms under which the partnership may be brought to an end and whether it is possible for a partner to be expelled, and, if so, in what circumstances. In the event of failure to deal with these aspects, it may be necessary to apply to the court to administer a dissolution of the partnership which will be lengthy and expensive for all the partners.

The partnership agreement should also deal with certain matters in relation to taxation, providing for the partnership to continue if this is advantageous from a tax point of view upon a change in personnel.

The agreement should also specify the way in which the records should be kept and the expenses which are to be regarded as expenses of the partnership. It should be remembered that there must be no transactions involving goodwill in the partnership of a medical practice. It is permissible to agree that a partner binds himself or herself out from an area for a period of time after retirement from the practice from an area. Restrictions of this type must be reasonable to be enforceable and specialist advice should be considered before drafting such a term to avoid the possibility that the term might subsequently be struck down in its entirety, thereby creating the opposite result to that intended.

Limitations regarding lists

Medical practice in partnership can also give rise to difficulties regarding share of workload and the lists system provides that not more than 4500 patients should be on the list of any one partner and that the average for the practice as a whole should not be more than 3500. Clearly, for each practitioner at the upper figure, other practitioners must operate with smaller than average lists. Further, if an assistant is employed, the number of patients may be increased by 2000 in respect of each assistant. Thus, if the practice is in a position to expand, there must be a considerable temptation to upgrade an assistant to partner. These figures are limits. In reality, average list sizes are more likely to be in the range of 1500–1800 patients.

Employees – statutory obligations on employment and termination

Over the last 25 years, employment law has been the subject of a long series of statutes which have had a substantial effect on the regulation of employment practices. The current governing statute as far as individual employment law is concerned is the Employment Rights Act 1996. This is a recent consolidation act. It seems likely that future political changes will result in at least substantial changes of detail if not wholesale further legislation in this field. In particular, legislation is likely to be introduced to implement the Working Hours Directive, which also has implications for holidays. Since a number of these rights are based upon directives of the European Union, there are a number of areas of uncertainty which may lead to appeals and references to the European Court. In particular these challenges to domestic legislation have been mounted in the context of qualifying periods for employment rights, both in terms of the duration of employment and the length of the qualifying working week. The only satisfactory way to approach these difficulties is to ensure that the practice has in place good employment practices and that those practices are observed by all members of staff, both the partnership and employees in relation to all employees whether part time or recently employed. Matters relating to sex and race discrimination are dealt with in a later section as is the topic of maternity.

It is important to remember that many of the decisions which the Industrial Tribunals face in dealing with employment law cases are based on a judicial analysis of the reasonableness of the actions of one of the parties. However, this question is normally considered in the framework of the Tribunal deciding whether the employer acted within a range of reasonable responses to a particular situation. For employers this is an important concept. The legislation itself is not inherently 'against' employers. In practice, the Tribunal is not rehearing, for example, a disciplinary investigation in order to reach its own conclusion. The Tribunal's task is to analyse whether the response was within a band of reasonable responses, after considering the way in which the employer reached the decision. It should also be emphasized that the legislation, as developed in cases, places great emphasis on two aspects of management conduct. These are the requirements for proper procedures and the observation of the tenets of natural justice.

At their simplest, the procedural requirements attached to disciplinary procedures should be indicated in the statement of terms and conditions of employment. These will normally stipulate in the context of conduct that there should be a series of warnings before dismissal is considered. There are no hard and fast rules about these matters, but it is normal for there to be an opportunity for at least one oral warning and one formal written warning before dismissal is considered. Similarly, procedures normally require that decisions relating to warnings are not taken in the heat of the moment, but after due consideration and after the employee has been given an opportunity to state his or her position and respond both to the allegation and in relation to the sanction. Further, in an ideal situation, investigation of a disciplinary offence should be undertaken by a different individual from the one deciding upon the appropriate sanction. As with all human relations, communication is the key concept. The employee who can establish that he or she was unaware that his or her dismissal was under consideration has a considerable advantage should the case come to a tribunal.

Key employment rights are shown in Box 7.2 (p. 140).

Turning to specific employment rights, a number should be mentioned.

1. Statement of terms and conditions of employment
This should be provided not later than 2 months after the beginning of employment. There is no express sanction or penalty if it is not given, although there has been recent adverse judicial comment in the context of a statement failing to contain a disciplinary proce-

Box 7.2
Key employment rights

1. To a statement of terms of employment.
2. To statutory minimum notice rights.
3. To an itemized pay statement.
4. Not to be dismissed for an inadmissible reason.
5. Not to be unfairly dismissed.
6. To a redundancy payment.
7. Not to be dismissed for pregnancy.
8. Maternity rights.
9. To bring a breach of contract claim.

dure and grievance procedure. It is important to remember that it is not a contract of employment. There is, therefore, no requirement to obtain the employee's agreement to its terms. Clearly, if it is issued within the appropriate time then the employer is giving a strong indication as to its view of the employment content at an early stage. It is customary, however, for employees to sign a copy to confirm that they have received the document. There is at present a part-timer exclusion for those working less than 8 hours a week, although it is desirable that all regular employees, for however short a time, should have a statement of this type. The statute prescribes certain terms which have to be included and, as might be expected, these include remuneration, hours of work, holidays, sick pay, pension entitlement, notice, disciplinary and grievance procedures and so forth. An employer who faces a Tribunal claim in respect of an employee who has not received a written statement is at an immediate disadvantage. In the absence of a statement, an employee can apply to a Tribunal to determine the terms applying.

2. Rights during notice

An employee has statutory entitlement to minimum notice of 1 week until the employee has worked for 2 years and thereafter 1 additional week for each year of employment up to a maximum of 12. During the period of notice, the employee has the benefit of certain rights unless they are contractually entitled to at least 1 week more notice than that prescribed by the statute. Most important is the right to receive payment during notice while incapable of work because of sickness or injury. If it is desired to exclude this provision, the employee must, therefore, be contractually entitled to at least 1 week more than the minimum under the provisions set out above.

3. Itemized pay statement

During employment, the employee enjoys a number of rights. Significantly these include the right to an itemized pay statement and the right to bring a claim in the event of an unlawful deduction in wages under Part II of the Employment Rights Act 1996 (formerly The Wages Act) or, in the event of breach of contract by the employer, under the contractual jurisdiction. This is now vested in the Industrial Tribunal. Sums should not be deducted from wages unless the employee has signed a written agreement approving the deductions.

4. *Inadmissible reason for dismissal*

During employment a number of rights are enjoyed without reference to a qualifying period. These include the right not to be dismissed for trade union activities nor to suffer a detriment short of dismissal for this reason. Also in this category is dismissal for certain health and safety reasons. Further an employee is entitled to bring a claim of unfair dismissal if the principal reason for the dismissal was that the employee asserted a statutory right.

5. *The right not to be unfairly dismissed*

If an employee has been working for 2 years he or she has a right to bring a claim of unfair dismissal. Provided the employer accepts that there was a dismissal, it is then for the employer to demonstrate the reason for that dismissal and that it was one of the potentially fair reasons. These are redundancy, conduct, the capability of the employee, breach of a statutory provision and, finally, what is called some other substantial reason ('SOSR'). The last mentioned is not a limitless category but has been recognized in a number of cases most notably where there is a reorganization of the business for bona fide commercial reasons. SOSR may also be an acceptable reason for dismissal where there has been a variation of terms of employment despite absence of a contractual right for the employer to vary terms.

The test of the fairness of the dismissal involves the employer demonstrating the reason for the dismissal and, thereafter, it is for the Tribunal hearing the case to decide whether the employer acted reasonably (i.e. within the band of reasonable responses) in treating the reasons shown for the dismissal as a sufficient reason for dismissing the employee.

One might ask how a Tribunal can possibly decide these issues. The Tribunal is intended to act as 'an industrial jury'. In other words, the chairman and the two members bring their experience of industrial relations viewed from both sides of the employment divide to their analysis of the issues and the way in which the case is presented.

If it is found that the employer dismissed an employee unfairly, the employee is entitled to an award or possibly an order for reinstatement. The financial award comprises a basic element which equates to the redundancy payment the employee would have been entitled to and a compensatory award to represent the financial loss which he or she has suffered as a result of the unfair dismissal. The award may be reduced if the employee contributed to the dismissal. Unlike awards in discrimination, these rights are subject to financial limits. Currently, the maximum amount of a weeks pay which can be taken into consideration for a basic award is £210 and the maximum compensatory award is £11 300. If the Tribunal orders reinstatement and the employer refuses to comply, then higher awards can be made.

6. The right to a redundancy payment

This accrues at different rates depending on the age of the employee. Under age 21, this is half a week's pay for each year of service, between 21 and 41 it is one week's pay for each year of service, and from age 41 to 64 it is one and a half week's wages for each year of service. The maximum number of years which can be claimed is 20 and the current maximum weekly pay to be taken into account is £210. The maximum is, therefore, £6300. The term redundancy has meaning in common parlance far beyond its technical meaning in a legal context. By statute, redundancy means that the employer's requirements for the employee or the type of work undertaken have ceased or diminished, or are expected to cease or diminish. A claim for a redundancy payment cannot be made unless the employee has been working for 2 years continuously with the employer or his or her predecessor. A redundancy payment cannot be claimed after normal retirement age, and there is an upper limit of 65 in any event with a tapering provision between 64 and 65.

7. The right not to be dismissed as a result of pregnancy

There is no qualifying period for this and dismissal on these grounds is automatically unfair. It should be remembered that there are financial limits on the award which can be made in the event of dismissal for this reason whereas a dismissal as a result of sex discrimination does not carry an upper financial limit for the award.

8. Maternity

The rules regarding timing are extremely complex. At its simplest, all employees have the right to 14 weeks maternity leave and statutory maternity pay. Those who have 2 years service have a further right to return to work up to 29 weeks after the birth.

9. Contract claims

Finally, Tribunal jurisdiction has been extended to include contractual claims for breach of contract on the part of employers. The upper limit is £25 000 and the claim must be brought within 3 months of the date of termination of employment. The employer has a right to counterclaim if faced with a claim of this type.

*Discrimination –
sex, race,
maternity and
disability*

In addition to the specific claim of dismissal for a pregnancy-related reason, the concepts of sex discrimination and racial discrimination are wide ranging, and include direct and indirect discrimination. Indirect discrimination involves imposing a requirement that a racial group or sex has difficulty in satisfying. This field of the law should not be approached in a pedantic frame of mind as in the case of the apocryphal story of the employer who simply said 'please tell us what words we are not allowed to use this year'. Good practice requires a change in attitude. This is involved at every stage of the recruitment and employment process from the initial enquiry regarding availability of vacancies through the interviewing procedure, selection of employees, opportunities for promotion and circumstances giving rise to termination of employment.

In particular, the concept of sexual harassment can have extremely wide implications in the workplace and in the manner in which the environment is controlled. The sensibilities of employees have to be taken into account in the way in which their colleagues are required to behave. Employers are under an active obligation to prevent harassment and discrimination. There are no qualifying periods in relation to these claims and the size of the awards can be substantial. They can include damages for injury to feelings. As with termination of employment, there are codes of practice on dealing with the problems if they arise in the workplace, and it must be borne in mind that the employers are normally responsible for the actions of their employees who may be pursuing discriminatory conduct of one sort of another against other employees. One particularly sensitive area which should be noted is that of telephone enquiries in relation to job applications. It is prudent to ensure that trained staff who understand these issues take telephone calls from applicants responding to advertisements and even from applicants who apply after the post has been filled. Records should be kept to ensure that callers can be identified and the time at which calls were made is logged. It is also important to monitor the interviewing procedure so that it can be established that the same matrix of questions was asked of each applicant and that the answers were considered in an objective way. As with termination of employment, procedures are all important. An unexplained failure to follow procedure can lead to a Tribunal drawing an inference that there has been discrimination. These difficulties should never arise if those responsible keep adequate records of the way in which key employment decisions are reached.

On 2 December 1996, the Disability Discrimination Act came into force in relation to employment. This makes it unlawful to treat anyone with a disability less favourably than anyone else without justification and will have wide-ranging implications both in the employment context and within provisions regarding building design in view of the requirements to make alterations to premises.

Employers will, therefore, need to be vigilant to ensure that they are in a position to adjust to facilitate the disabled employee and aware of the detailed provisions of the Act and Codes of Practice made under it.

There is an exemption for employers with fewer than 20 employees.

Termination of employment and dissolution of partnership

Termination of employment

A termination of employment checklist is shown in Box 7.3.

Termination of employment should in every case, regardless of employee's length of service, be undertaken after due considera-tion and with courage and humanity. If the relationship has not worked out, it is better that it should be brought to an end in an open, frank and courteous fashion. Many employers will say that it was imperative that employment be brought to an end at 5 o'clock on Friday with payment in lieu of notice because of their fear that the dismissed employee would 'poison' the other staff. That is a decision which should not be taken lightly as the manner of dismissal, while only rarely having an impact on the amount of any compensation, may be a deciding factor in whether the disap-pointed employee brings a Tribunal claim at all. Considering termination of employment, the following checklist should be utilized and the key points are considered as follows:

1. Is there a contract of employment or statement of terms? If not, is there any explanation?
2. Procedure. Is the proposed reason for dismissal sufficient to justify immediate dismissal and have the appropriate prelimin-ary warnings already been given?
3. Is the reason proposed for the dismissal the true reason? If a different reason is found to have been the underlying reason at the Tribunal, it is difficult to envisage that the dismissal will be accepted as fair.
4. Have any procedural requirements in connection with the dismissal itself been undertaken. In a dismissal for dishonesty, has such investigation as a reasonable employer would require been undertaken?

Box 7.3
Termination of employment checklist

1. Is there a contract of employment?
2. Have all warning procedures been followed?
3. What is the true reason for the dismissal?
4. What are the correct procedures for the disciplinary action?
5. Is dismissal the appropriate sanction?
6. Has the employee been offered a right of appeal?
7. Is it proposed to replace the employee?

5. Is dismissal the appropriate action? Is there any prospect that the employee might prefer to resign to avoid the stigma of dismissal in the search for new employment?
6. Has the employee been offered a right of appeal? Is it to be a complete rehearing or just a check on formalities?
7. Is it proposed to replace the employee? Is this consistent with the reason for the dismissal, e.g. redundancy?

Dissolution of partnership

1. If the agreement is carefully drafted then a retirement or departure should have been planned in advance. In particular issues such as sale of the outgoing partner's share, continuation for tax purposes and use of the premises will be covered.
2. If the agreement does not cover these aspects, then the partners should endeavour to reach agreement normally with at least one set of professional advisers. When agreement is reached, it should be considered in the framework of a dissolution agreement.
3. In the absence of agreement and in the absence of an arbitration provision, an action will be brought in the court for dissolution. This will normally involve ruling on the terms of partnership, if these are disputed, and providing for an account to be taken in accordance with those terms. The court may then order payments to be made pursuant to the account.

RELATIONSHIP WITH PATIENTS

Consent to treatment

A checklist for consent to treatment is shown in Box 7.4.

In the leading case of Sidaway v Board of Governors of the Bethlem Royal Hospital and the Maudsley Hospital (1985), the House of Lords rejected the concept of informed consent as part of English Law and in effect accepted what is known as the 'Bolam' test (see below) with its reliance on an established body of medical opinion as justification for particular practices in the context of consent.

The present position is that the doctor must warn the patient of material risks so as not to vitiate any consent which he or she may

Box 7.4
Consent checklist

1. Has the patient asked about risks? If so, answer truthfully.
2. Is a warning likely to be detrimental to the patient's health?
3. If so, consider warning if there are substantial risks of grave consequences.
4. Consider whether *the patient* would regard a risk as significant.
5. Obtain consent after warning as appropriate.

obtain to the treatment. If the treatment is carried out without consent, then there is a danger that the patient may pursue an action in battery against the practitioner. The doctor is under an obligation to warn the patient of risks inherent in the treatment. The duty is confined to material risk. This is tested by analysing whether a court would be satisfied that a reasonable person in the patient's position would be likely to attach significance to the risk.

Even if the risk is material, the doctor will not be liable if upon a reasonable assessment of the condition, he or she takes the view that a warning would be detrimental to the patient's health. There is also judicial opinion to the effect that, in certain circumstances, treatment might involve such a substantial risk of grave consequences that, notwithstanding the view of a responsible body of medical opinion, a patient should be told of the risk as no prudent medical person should refrain from telling the patient of that type of risk. The position may also be altered if the patient specifically asks about risks. A doctor is under a duty to answer truthfully and as fully as the question requires, if the patient poses the question.

Negligence – liability in tort
Medical practitioners have a duty of care in tort to their patients. There is no requirement for any contractual relationship with the patient. The duty of care is imposed even when the services are given gratuitously. There can be no liability for failing to treat a patient who refuses consent who is adult and of sound mind. A duty of care is also owed to the unborn.

The standard of skill and care is based in modern law on the case of Bolam v Friern Hospital Management Committee (1957). Shortly stated, the test is the standard of the ordinary skilled person exercising and professing to have the special medical skill in question. Negligence means failure to act in accordance with the standards of a reasonably competent medical person at the time. There may be one or more perfectly proper standards and, if the practitioner conforms with one of the accepted standards, then he or she is not negligent.

If the care falls short of the accepted standard, the question of causation of loss arises. Liability is established if the negligent act caused or materially contributed to the injury. The patient recovers his or her damages in full if he or she can show that there was a material contribution regardless of the fact that there may have been other material factors contributing at the same time. If the patient is suing for the loss of a chance (e.g. of recovery to good health), then he or she must merely show that there was a prospect in excess of 50% of the injury not occurring to recover in full for the loss of that chance.

Finally, it should be mentioned that there are a number of difficult reported decisions in connection with the way in which the chain of causation operates after a negligent act. These deal with the remoteness of the consequences which can be laid at the door of a practitioner who has failed to observe the appropriate standard when there has been an intervening event.

Children – Gillick competence and consent

Under the Children Act 1989 a parent may consent to medical treatment on behalf of a child where the child is incompetent. Further, under Section 3(5) of the Act, the person who has care of the child may do what is reasonable in all the circumstances of the case for the purposes of safeguarding or promoting the child's welfare. There is some debate as to whether this section would extend to consenting to medical treatment. Further, the court may consent under its wardship jurisdiction or under Section 8 of the Act on behalf of the child. The person consenting on behalf of the child must act in the best interests of the child and a parent's right to consent must be exercised in accordance with this principle otherwise it can be challenged. In similar terms, the court exercises a power to authorize medical treatment on an incompetent adult. In the case of emergencies, a patient who is temporarily unconscious and unable to give consent should be able to receive treatment from a practitioner who is free from threat of action for trespass to the patient provided the treatment is both necessary and cannot be reasonably delayed. Similar principles apply in the case of the temporarily incompetent, while in the case of the permanently incompetent patient action can be properly taken to preserve life, health or well-being provided the need for care is obvious. The doctor must act in the best interests of the patient.

To what extent can a competent child refuse medical treatment? After the case of Gillick v West Norfolk and Wisbech AHA (1986), it was recognized that a minor child could be competent in law to make his or her own decisions provided he or she has a sufficient understanding and intelligence to enable him or her to understand fully what is proposed. Despite this House of Lords decision, the Court of Appeal has subsequently increased the complexity of this field by ruling that, although Gillick allows a competent child to consent to treatment without the possibility of being overruled by the parents, refusal of treatment by a competent child does not have the same force and can be overruled by the parents or the courts.

Vicarious liability for acts of employees

A partner in general practice is liable not only for the acts of his or her partners but also for the negligence of the partnership staff. There is, therefore, a liability for members of staff performing functions for the practice. An employee is not liable for the negligent acts of his or her fellow employees.

Case study – the receptionist

In the case of Lobley v Going and others (1985), a 22-month-old child suffering with a sore throat was brought to the surgery at 5 p.m. The receptionist was told that the child had difficulty breathing and the parents were asked to wait. The parents wished to take the child to see the doctor as soon as possible because of his breathing and the receptionist told them that she would see what could be done. After 15 minutes, the parents insisted on the child being seen immediately. When the doctor saw the child, an ambulance was called but unfortunately the child suffered an hypoxic interlude. At hospital, he suffered cardiac arrest and irreparable brain damage. In this case, it was held that a receptionist could be guilty of negligence in failing to inform the doctor immediately if a child with respiratory difficulties was brought to the surgery. However, it was not sufficient for the parents to indicate a measure of concern and expect the receptionist to enquire of them regarding the condition of the child. The case had not been referred to as an emergency when the parents arrived at the surgery, and the practice was held not to have been negligent.

Access to medical records There are four relevant statutes to consider. These are summarized in Box 7.5 and considered in detail below.

Box 7.5
Medical records:
relevant statutes

1. Access to Health Records Act 1990
   – Gives access to non-computerized records after 1 November 1991
2. Data Protection Act 1984
   – Access to computerized records
3. Access to Medical Reports Act 1988
   – Access to employment and insurance reports
4. Supreme Court Act 1981 Section 33
   – Pre-action discovery

1. Access to Health Records Act 1990
A patient has a right to non-computerized health records for which an application can be made under the Act. Inspection must be allowed and copies must be supplied within 40 days. In respect of records less than 40 days old, inspection and supply should be provided within 21 days. Access is provided in connection with post-1 November 1991 information. There is an exception in relation to records produced for children. Here the holder has to be satisfied that the child is capable of understanding the nature of the application. Either the child must consent or the holder must be satisfied that the child is incapable of understanding the nature of the application and that access would be in the child's best interests.

In connection with the records of a deceased person, if a note has been made at the deceased' request that he or she did not wish access to be given, this is a ground for refusing.

There is also a general exception under Section 5(1) where the information would be likely to cause serious harm to the physical or mental health of the patient or any other individual. In this case, disclosure need not be given and it can be refused where it might lead to the identification of an informant concerning the patient, unless the individual has consented. An application can be made to correct inaccurate records or the practitioner can record the perceived inaccuracy notified by the patient.

2. The Data Protection Act 1984
This is part of the general right of access to computerized records. There is a limitation by statutory instrument of 1987 in the case of serious harm to the physical or mental health of the patient or revelation of the identity of an informant.

3. The Access to Medical Reports Act 1988
Access is available to medical reports provided for the purposes of employment and insurance. This will not generally result in disclosure of medical notes. Again there is an exception under Section 7 in the case of serious harm to the physical or mental health of the individual or of others, or revelation of the identity of an informer.

4. Pre-action discovery under the Supreme Court Act 1981 Section 33
This allows the plaintiff access to medical and nursing notes and ancillary materials so that they can be seen before action has been commenced. It remains important because it is not subject to the exceptions referred to above. It is again available against third parties who are not potential parties to the litigation.

It may be a daunting prospect but all notes should be written on the assumption that they may at some stage come into the hands of the patient or their legal advisors in a hostile context.

Confidentiality   The Hippocratic Oath states:

> *whatsoever things I see or hear concerning the life of men, in my attendance on the sick or even apart therefrom, which ought not to be noised abroad, I will keep silence thereon, counting such things to be as sacred secrets.*

Information is confidential if it is supplied in circumstances where the recipient has notice or is aware that the information is confidential. The duty of confidence has been generally assumed in the few reported cases in which it has been considered. There is advice given by the General Medical Council (October, 1995) in the booklet 'Confidentiality' forming part of the set 'Duties of a Doctor'. It is the doctor's duty strictly to observe the rule of professional secrecy by refraining from disclosing voluntarily to any third party information about a patient which he has learned directly or indirectly in his or her professional capacity as a registered practitioner. There are certain statutory endorsements of this obligation in the context of, for example, venereal diseases and embryology. Confidential information may be received from third parties whether they are lay persons or health care professionals.

Further difficulties arise in the case of children. One view is that, if the child is incompetent to give consent, then he or she cannot expect to form a relationship of confidentiality with the doctor. It may be that capacity and competence will not arrive together at a particular instant in time. There may be a series of points where the child becomes entitled to greater confidentiality as his or her competence increases. There is also the question of an overriding obligation of disclosure if it is in the best interests of the child, for example, in compelling circumstances such as physical or sexual abuse.

In the case of incompetent adults it would appear to follow that these individuals can never form a confidential relationship, although disclosure would appear to require justification for disclosure in the best interests of the incompetent adult on an analogy with children.

The position of confidence in relation to deceased patients is more difficult. Action is not possible in defamation on behalf of the deceased's estate. A similar position may arise in relation to a breach of confidence in the absence of a demonstrable detriment to the estate. However, a practitioner disclosing in these circumstances might encounter difficulties in other directions. For example, if financial gain was achieved through misuse of confidential information, the estate might raise an argument in unjust enrichment and even if the disclosure was not for such gain it might be termed frivolous and lead to possible application of professional sanctions.

The broad obligation of confidentiality is varied both in circumstances of individual consent and in a number of statutory instances. There may also be arguments relating to public interest justification for disclosure. These subjects are outside the scope of this work.

THE UNDERLYING LEGAL FRAMEWORK TO GENERAL PRACTICE

This framework is summarized in Box 7.6 (opposite).

1. Definition of a registered medical practitioner

A registered medical practitioner is defined in Section 3 of the Medical Act 1983 as someone holding a primary UK qualification who has passed a qualifying examination and satisfied the requirements as to experience. Provisional registration arises in the case of

Box 7.6
Legal framework to
general practice

1. Definition of a registered medical practitioner.
2. Application for inclusion on the list of practitioners.
3. Scope of service.
4. Terms of service.
5. Medical services.
6. New patients.
7. Consultations.
8. Appointments.
9. General.
10. Records.
11. Fundholding.
12. Practice-based complaints procedures.

graduates from medical school to allow them to fulfil the training requirement in a resident medical capacity. Anyone who falsely pretends to take the title of physician, doctor or the like is liable to a fine on conviction and no one can recover a charge for medical advice unless they are fully registered.

Originally, family practitioner committees, subsequently family health service authorities and more recently health authorities have a statutory duty to provide personal medical services in their localities. This body is referred to as 'the authority' in the remainder of the section.

2. Application for inclusion on the list of general medical practitioners   A doctor who wishes to be included on the list must make an application for inclusion to the authority. The primary regulations governing the list are the 1992 National Health Service (General Medical Services) Regulations as subsequently amended. When a doctor applies, a report must be made to the Medical Practices Committee, which determines the application. Conditions can be imposed. Regulation 15 provides that a doctor can be included in the list as a full-time doctor, which is for more than 26 hours per week, a three-quarter time doctor, between 19 and 26 hours, and half-time doctor, between 13 and 19 hours, or a job-sharing doctor who with another doctor is available for 26 hours a week. There is a further class of restricted doctors whose obligation is to provide services during the number of hours specified in the application. Conditions may also be attached in relation to the provision of services in specified parts of the locality of the authority. If there is an application for variation of conditions representations are made and are passed to the Medical Practices Committee. There can be an appeal to the Secretary of State against decisions of this committee.

3. Scope of service   Regulation 3 sets out the scope and terms of services involved in general medical services. These include all the necessary and appropriate personal medical services usually provided by general medical practitioners. Reference is also made to child health surveillance services, contraceptive services, maternity medical services and minor surgery services.

4. The terms of service   The arrangements for provision of service refer to Schedule 2 of the Regulations which sets out in detail the terms of service. Particular points to note are that, under paragraph 3, the degree of skill, knowledge and care required is defined as that which general practitioners as a class may reasonably be expected to exercise. The doctor's patients are defined in paragraph 4 and, in addition to those on his or her list, these include those for whom he or she is acting as a deputy for another doctor. During hours arranged with the authority any person whose own doctor has been relieved of responsibility during those hours becomes a patient. A doctor may accept a person on his or her list as a patient if the person is eligible to be accepted by him or her. A doctor is required to give the authority 8 days notice that he or she wishes to have a person removed from his or her list. Special provisions for removal apply in the case of a patient who has been violent to the doctor.

5. Medical services   Paragraph 12 provides that a doctor shall render to his or her patients all necessary and appropriate medical services. These are defined in paragraph 12. They include advice in connection with the patients' general health, diet, exercise, use of tobacco, consumption of alcohol, and misuse of drugs or solvents. The patient is to be offered consultations and, where appropriate, physical examination for the purpose of identifying or reducing risk of disease or injury. Appropriate vaccinations are to be offered in relation to certain specified diseases and arrangements are to be made for the referral of patients to other services. The services also include giving advice to enable patients to avail themselves of services provided by the local social services authority.

6. New patients   Within 28 days of acceptance of a new patient on to the doctor's list the doctor is to invite the patient to attend a consultation. At that time, the doctor is to seek details of the patient's medical history and that of his or her family and offer physical examination. It is clearly intended by the regulations that there should be an assessment at this stage regarding the patient's continuing medical care. Invitation to this consultation is to be made in writing or, if made orally, confirmed in writing. If the doctor becomes aware the patient no longer resides at the address given, the authority is to be informed. The consultation need not be offered to children under 5 or patients who were on the list of a partner and who received an initial consultation in the 12 months prior to the date of acceptance.

If a doctor assumes responsibility for a list on succession to a practice or otherwise becomes responsible for a large number of new patients, he or she can apply to defer this obligation for a period not exceeding 2 years. Such an application must state the doctor's proposals by reference to particular classes of patients and should be determined by the authority within 2 months.

7. Consultations   Patients aged between 16 and 75 who have not been seen within a 3-year period are entitled to request a consultation to assess their needs for general medical services. If aged over 75, each patient should be invited to a consultation once in each period of 12 months beginning on 1 April in each year.

8. Appointments   Persons who attend at the practice during the hours approved by the authority (unless they attend without appointment when an appointments system is in operation) are entitled to be seen and treated. If the doctor is entitled to refuse to see them because they have failed to observe the appointment systems, the doctor can refuse provided the health of the patient will not be jeopardized and the patient is offered an appropriate appointment to attend. A doctor is required to take steps to ensure that patients are not refused treatment without his or her knowledge.

9. General   The Regulations also deal with absences, deputies, assistants and partners. The authority is entitled to inspect the premises. Before employing an assistant, the practitioner must satisfy himself or herself that the employee is suitably qualified and competent to discharge his or her duties. The doctor is obliged to afford employees reasonable opportunities to undertake training to maintain their competence. The area of practice cannot be changed without the consent of the authority.

New Regulations provide for cases where practitioners are suspended or disqualified by NHS Tribunal and the provision of services to suspended doctors' patients.

10. Records   The doctor should keep adequate records and forward them to the authority on request as soon as possible and at the latest within 14 days of being informed by the authority of the death of a patient. If the doctor becomes aware of the death other than from the authority, the records must be forwarded within 1 month. Annual reports have to be made to the authority.

11. Fundholding   Under the National Health Service and Community Care Act 1990 Sections 14–17, practices can be organized as fundholding practices. These practices are entitled to purchase services within the internal market of the NHS. Recognition is on application and satisfaction of certain conditions contained in regulations made in 1990.

12. Practice-based complaints procedures

On 1 April 1996 it became a requirement of the terms of service for a doctor to establish a practice-based complaints procedure. Requirements for the procedure are established, with provisions for recording and acknowledging complaints. Complaints must be properly investigated. The result of the investigation and the conclusion should be issued within 10 days of receipt by the person responsible. Doctors must inform patients about the procedure. They must also cooperate in the Health Authority Complaints Procedure (see page 156).

THE REGULATORS, PROFESSIONAL, HEALTH SERVICE AND OTHERS

The General Medical Council

A summary of the Committees making up the regulatory function of the General Medical Council (GMC) is shown in Box 7.7.

The GMC is the professional body exercising control over standards of professional and private conduct of medical practitioners. Section 36 of the Medical Act 1983 allows the GMC through its committee to erase a name from the register or suspend for a period of 12 months or to make registration conditional on compliance with specified requirements to protect the public. These powers arise in the event of conviction for a criminal offence or in the event that the Professional Conduct Committee adjudges the practitioner to have been guilty of serious professional misconduct. Guidance on the way in which these powers are operated is contained in the booklet *Duties of a Doctor – Good Medical Practice* published by the GMC in October 1995.

There is a Preliminary Proceedings Committee which selects the cases to be referred for enquiry by the Professional Conduct Committee and both Committees are advised on questions of law by a Legal Assessor. Convictions of doctors are normally reported to the Council by the Police and, unless they relate to minor motoring or other trivial offences, are normally referred to the Preliminary Proceedings Committee.

Matters of serious professional misconduct may be referred to the Committee by individual doctors or members of the public. These references must generally be supported by evidence in the form of affidavits. In some cases the Council's Solicitor may be asked to make enquiries to establish the facts. The Preliminary Proceedings Committee may decide to deal with the matter by way of a letter of warning or advice, and the case is not then pursued. If the Committee feels that there may be a physical or mental

Box 7.7
GMC Committees

- ◆ The Preliminary Proceedings Committee.
- ◆ The Professional Conduct Committee.
- ◆ The Health Committee.
- ◆ The Committee on Professional Performance.

condition causing the problem, the case may be referred to the Health Committee instead of the Professional Conduct Committee. If a case is referred to either the Health Committee or the Professional Conduct Committee, a preliminary interim suspension may be made for a period not exceeding 2 months. No such order should be made unless the doctor has been offered an opportunity to appear and be heard in relation to the order being made.

In addition to the other powers mentioned above, the Committee also has a power at the conclusion of an enquiry to postpone its determination. This is normally done to allow the names of colleagues to be provided to give information regarding the doctor's conduct since the previous hearing. In some cases a subsequent period of postponement may be imposed if the Committee does not feel able to conclude the case after replies are received from referees.

The difficult element of this jurisdiction is to identify what exactly is meant by 'serious professional misconduct'. All practitioners will be concerned to identify where the distinction is to be drawn between professional misconduct and medical negligence. The GMC is only concerned with matters which give rise to actions in negligence when the conduct has involved such a disregard of professional responsibility to patients or professional duties as to raise a question of serious professional misconduct. An example given is a doctor endangering the welfare of patients by persisting to engage in unsupervised practice of a branch of medicine without having the appropriate knowledge and skill and without having acquired the necessary experience. There is no doubt that since 1979 the GMC has become more concerned with errors of clinical judgement. Examples of serious professional misconduct include neglect or disregard of personal responsibilities to patients, abuse of professional privileges or skills and personal behaviour which is derogatory to the reputation of the medical profession. In the publication *Duties of a Doctor* (GMC, 1995) the GMC provides guidance on good medical practice, advertising, HIV and AIDS, and confidentiality.

Under the Medical (Professional Performance) Act 1995, Parliament has allowed the GMC to establish a new Committee to deal with the unfortunate small number of medical practitioners whose standards from time to time fall below that which the patients have the right to expect. In addition to the Medical Committee and the Professional Conduct Committee, there will now be the Committee on Professional Performance Committee to ensure that doctors maintain their competence. The arrangements are to be implemented on 1 September 1997 and allow conditions to be imposed on, or the suspension of, a doctor's registration in the event of serious deficiencies in standards of professional performance. The power to strike off the register is not included, although there may be indefinite suspension. There will be procedures to provide for screening of complaints of this type and assessment of performance before a reference is made to the Committee. The GMC has the power to make rules to be approved by the Privy Council.

The new NHS complaints procedure The National Health Service (Function of Health Authorities) (Complaints) Regulations 1996 came into force on 1 April 1996, and confer on health authorities the function of establishing and operating procedures for dealing with complaints about family health service practitioners in accordance with directions made by the Secretary of State under the National Health Service Act 1977. On 28 March 1996, a direction was made setting up the new procedure and the following points represent a brief outline of the new procedure.

Complaints are not appropriate where the complainant states that he or she intends to pursue a remedy by legal proceedings. The health authorities are required to appoint a complaints manager, and a complaint can be made by patients or former patients of a practitioner or on behalf of a child or by a relative of an incapable adult. A complaint can be made on behalf of a deceased former patient.

The complaint must be made within a basic period of 6 months from the date of the treatment or 6 months from the date of the complainant's knowledge, with an overall time limit of 12 months. There is a discretion to extend the time limit. If there is a refusal to allow an extension of time, there is an appeal to the Health Service Commissioner.

The initial procedure after making a complaint is that the matter is referred to conciliation, in the event that the person making the complaint cannot reasonably be expected to make a complaint directly to a 'practice-based complaints procedure'. Conciliation is also available in the course of an investigation under a practice-based complaints procedure. If the complainant is dissatisfied with the outcome of a practice-based complaints procedure, they can subsequently be referred to conciliation.

If still dissatisfied, the complainant should complain to the complaints manager. Every health authority must make arrangements to appoint a convener whose job is to make arrangements to resolve complaints where the complainant is dissatisfied with the outcome of conciliation or the practice-based complaints procedure. A panel may then be appointed to conduct an independent investigation. The complainant has 21 days to ask the convener to investigate. The convener has to receive a complaint in writing setting out the complaint before he or she can proceed and the statement has then to be referred to the practitioner who is the subject of the complaint. The convener must then decide whether further action can be taken by the practitioner to satisfy the complainant and whether no further benefit would be achieved by appointing an independent panel.

If the convener decides to appoint a panel, he or she should also ask the health authority to consider whether the matter should be referred to any of the professional regulatory bodies or the NHS tribunal or the police. It may also be referred back for further investigation or conciliation. If the matter is referred to a professional regulatory body, the convener ceases to take any action.

The convener is required before taking decisions regarding the panel to consult, in the cases of clinical judgment, with a person from a list appointed by the Secretary of State and in every case with a person from a list nominated by the Secretary of State. After he or she has made his or her decision, the convener specifies the matters to be investigated by the panel or notifies the complainant that he or she has determined that it is not appropriate to appoint a panel and indicates that the complainant has a right to complain to the Health Service Commissioner. The Health Service Commissioner can overrule the decision not to investigate.

The panel which investigates is a three-member group consisting of the convener and two persons from a list of persons nominated by the Secretary of State. One of these is the independent lay chairman. It may also be necessary for assessors to be appointed when issues of clinical judgment arise. The panel can govern its own procedure and the participants can be interviewed together or separately. The complainant and any other person interviewed may be accompanied by another person provided that they do not act as advocate if they are legally qualified.

The panel then reports on the findings of fact it has made, its opinion and reasons and the report of the assessors if appropriate. There is also provision for complaints about the use of the allotted sum under Section 15 of the National Health Service and Community Care Act 1990. The report of the panel can include suggestions which will improve the services provided by practitioners. It may not suggest disciplinary procedures. There is an appeal from the finding of the panel to the Health Services Commissioner (the Ombudsman).

Community health councils These are established to represent the interests of the public in the health service for the area. They review the operation of the health service and make recommendations to the authority. They are consulted on substantial variations to services. They can inspect premises controlled by the health service. The council can help the individual patient to complain, through the NHS, the Ombudsman or by legal action.

The Patients Association This association is funded by private subscription, donations and a government grant. It campaigns for improved relations between patients and others in medical practice.

CONCLUSION This chapter gives an indication of a number of important areas where common law and statutory jurisdictions regulate both business activities and the way in which medicine is practised. While an unduly detailed appreciation of the legal issues may be a drawback in general practice, there is no doubt that an overall understanding of the issues both in business law and in medical law is not only beneficial to the practice but essential in avoiding problems before they arise.

SUMMARY

The key points in this chapter can be summarized as follows:

♦ All business arrangements benefit from a clear basis of agreement negotiated freely between parties who understand the risks and benefits of the activities on which they are about to embark.
♦ In dealing with employees, there is now a significant code of employment law which requires employees to be treated with humanity and dignity, and this approach will benefit the relationship both for the employers and employees.
♦ Termination of employment and dissolution of partnership are complex areas that are to be approached with extreme care.
♦ Medical negligence is measured predominantly against the standards of practice accepted by a significant body of colleagues.
♦ Issues relating to consent, confidentiality and medical records should be carefully considered, and the practice should provide guidelines for safe operation for the partners and staff.
♦ The underlying framework of the practice is ultimately a matter of statutory instrument and, therefore, a matter of legislation. There is no contractual relationship with the patient.
♦ In addition to the practitioner's own medical professional body, there are also statutory supervision, community health council supervision and patients' pressure groups to consider.

FURTHER READING

♦ Perrins, B. (ed.) (1997) *Harvey on Industrial Relations and Employment Law*. Butterworths, London.

The definitive employment law encyclopaedia, in four loose leaf volumes. This is a must helpful, but detailed, specialist publication.

♦ Kennedy, I., Grubb, A. (eds) (1994) *Medical Law*, 2nd edn. Butterworths, London.

A stimulating academic textbook, with helpful extracts from interesting materials and analytical argument.

♦ Lewis, C.J. (1995) *Medical Negligence*, 3rd edn. Tolley, Croydon.

A practical handbook both in relation to the legal issues and also on the day-to-day steps involved in the conduct of litigation.

♦ I'anson Banks, R.C. (ed.) (1995) *Lindley and Banks on Partnership*, 17th edn. Sweet & Maxwell, London.

A practitioner's legal textbook addressing partnership law generally.

STATUTES   Partnership Act 1890. HMSO.
QUOTED   Race Relations Act 1968. HMSO.
Sex Discrimination Act 1975. HMSO.
National Health Service Act 1977. HMSO.
Supreme Court Act 1981. HMSO.
Medical Act 1983. HMSO.
Data Protection Act 1984. HMSO.
Access to Medical Reports Act 1988. HMSO.
Children Act 1989. HMSO.
National Health Service and Community Care Act 1990. HMSO.
Access to Health Records Act 1990. HMSO.
Medical (Professional Performance) Act 1995. HMSO.
Disability Discrimination Act 1996. HMSO.
Employment Rights Act 1996. HMSO.

REFERENCES   Directions to Health Authorities about dealing with complaints about
Regulations   Family Health Services Practitioners. HMSO.
National Health Service (Function of Health Authorities) Complaints
Regulations 1996. HMSO.
National Health Service (General Medical Services) Regulations 1992 (as
amended). HMSO.

Other publications   General Medical Council (1995), *Duties of a Doctor - Good Medical
Practice.* GMC, London.
General Medical Council (1997), *Performance Procedures, A Summary of
Current Proposals* - 3rd March. GMC, London.

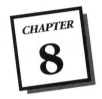

EFFECTIVE FINANCIAL MANAGEMENT

CHAPTER 8

Laurence Slavin

OBJECTIVES

- ◆ To show the importance of effective financial management within the current changes facing general practice partnerships.

- ◆ To understand the principles of financial management to control and manage financial affairs.

- ◆ To provide practical guidance on the purpose and components of the annual accounts.

- ◆ To understand financial monitoring together with the key financial indicators of practice performance and their role in financial planning.

INTRODUCTION

General practitioners in the UK provide services for the National Health Service (NHS), as opposed to being given a contract of service similar to that which their hospital colleagues are employed by. The subtle difference between a contract for services and a contract of service enables the general practitioner (GP) to have the independent contractor status which gives the GP the right to be self-employed, and the right to manage his or her own affairs (although perhaps to an increasingly lesser extent – see later). The GP is responsible for employing staff, controlling the finances, and has some choice in choosing how and what services are provided to patients.

GPs were given a new contract in 1990 that changed two aspects of their work. Firstly, it changed many of the items for which GPs were paid, introducing cash-limited funds and targets to be achieved but, more importantly, it changed the attitude of many GPs to the responsibilities of running a business. Before the new contract in 1990, discussions of money were in many cases looked on with disdain, but the targeting mechanism and ever-changing rules and goalposts have forced GPs to become more proactive in the management of their business. Ironically, under the old contract, 40% of the target gross income was intended to be paid by way of capitation, while under the new contract, as much as 60% of the intended gross income should be paid by capitation. The important difference is that the additional 40% non-capitation is more difficult to attain then the 60% was under the old contract.

The GP remuneration system is essentially a cost plus contract. A GP's remuneration is broken down into directly reimbursing some expenses, indirectly reimbursable expenses and setting out the intended average net income (IANI). The level of rise of this income is set each year by the government after they take advice from the Doctors' and Dentists' Review Body (DDRB). The DDRB obtains its information from a variety of sources. The main provider is the Inland Revenue, which conducts an annual survey of GPs' accounts extracting information and passing this on to a technical sub-committee of members of the Department of Health and the British Medical Association (BMA) which, in turn, advises the DDRB. This process is essentially working in arrears and is also used to confirm whether GPs have been overpaid or underpaid in the past, and is part of the clawback mechanism. The Inland Revenue is revising the manner in which the self-employed are taxed. The change to a current year basis, and the fact that GPs will assess their own tax liability without the Inland Revenue having sight of the accounts, means that the accounts review process will have to be amended. This process means that, as yet, income is set nationally with little local variation. This may change.

The present The current system, while attempting to maintain a GP's net income, has a number of inherent weaknesses. These can be summarized (see Box 8.1).

Box 8.1
Current system
weaknesses

1. Lack of 'accounts' standard or format.
2. Income inequality.
3. Income limit.
4. National pay setting.

1. Lack of standard 'accounts'
There is a necessary reliance on the Inland Revenue who in turn rely on the accountants' information. There is no prescriptive format to prepare the accounts and vital information can be omitted or hidden in the accounts. There is no audit of the information provided. This makes it particularly difficult for the Department of Health to announce, and for GPs to accept, that their evidence suggests GPs have been overpaid for a particular year.

2. Income inequality

In setting an intended average net remuneration, most GPs will have net income in a range £5000 either side of IANI. This does not properly reflect the difference between the deserving and non-deserving GPs, and, in turn, is one of the factors that has reduced morale and led some GPs to call for an end to the independent contractor status.

3. Income limit

The new contract is made up of a number of items for which GPs receive payment. The effect of the changes to the contract has been to limit the amount of income that can be earned (note the change in health promotion clinics from a per clinic basis to a set payment in a banding structure) and, as GPs have been more successful, so their intended level of income is set on the basis that more and more GPs will achieve all the targets and maximize the sources of income. There is less scope to generate further income and, therefore, greater emphasis on achieving all targets simply to be an average earning practice. Perversely, the greater the success, the more the urge seems to be from the DDRB to increase the targets, compounding the problem.

4. National pay setting

The new contract is centrally priced and no local circumstances are taken into account. A practice situated next to or near a local clinic will find it difficult, if not impossible, to persuade parents that their children should be immunized in the practice rather than at the clinic, which reduces the target payments to the practice. A practice may have a difficult group of patients refusing smears or immunizations which will directly affect their income. They may spend more time attempting to persuade the patients to attend the surgery than they would immunizing or smearing the patients. Deprivation payment is intended to compensate those practices in deprived areas from an inherent inability to maximize their income. It is not uncommon to find so-called deprived practices achieving all their targets, boosting their income above IANI. There needs to be some local flexibility in setting pay, a factor condoned in part of the 1995 Review Body report on doctors and dentists remuneration commenting on local flexibility (para 152).

At the same time the Department of Health brought in the new contract in 1990, it also introduced the concept of fundholding (formerly, and perhaps more accurately, known as budget holding). For the first time, GPs were empowered with some financial responsibility for negotiating hospital contracts for their referrals, a drugs budget for their prescribing, and securing a budget for staff costs. The financial control of fundholding is a specialized area, with regular audits and purpose-built software, and out of the scope of this section.

The GP partnership – the traditional approach
Some mention should be given to the way GPs work together. In the vast majority of cases, where more than one GP works together, they will work in partnership. This is very different from other professions where a minority of qualified accountants and solicitors will find themselves in partnership, but will have careers as managers. When other professions take new partners, it will be after a long probation period which perhaps can take up to 10 years before an equity partnership is offered. In general practice, the partner can be offered equity after a few months. Finding an inappropriate partner can be an expensive business and, while the advice and direction for this issues is outside the scope of this book, the financial costs can be considerable.

The future The position of the GP in the NHS is pivotal, the gatekeeper into secondary care, and constantly attracts interest from the Secretary of State for Health at the time. The GPs' contract is likely to change substantially in the next 5 years. Demand for a salaried service from the GPs themselves could be an option, the ever-decreasing ability to match health resources with demand will most probably involve GPs in the rationing process all within a framework of local pay negotiation and local accountability.

PRINCIPLES OF All businesses need to control and manage their financial affairs.
FINANCIAL General practice is no different, although there are still a number of
MANAGEMENT GPs who refuse to accept they are conducting a business and, invariably, it is these GPs who will fail to maximize their profits or, worse, fail to generate sufficient income to meet their personal and practice needs.

It is often stated that it is not possible to predict and budget GPs' income owing to ever-changing rules and moving goalposts (e.g. changes in payments for health promotion clinics), but it needs to be remembered that budgeting is not an exact science, it is an attempt to predict future income and expenses. The income and expenses of general practice are far easier to predict than most other businesses as patient list sizes rarely change dramatically, there is a set fee-scale and few changes occur without prior consultation.

Budgeting and Forecasts are a prediction of likely events and need to be updated
forecasting on a regular basis.

Profits forecast and There are two practical techniques that practices should perform, a
cash-flow forecast profits forecast and a cash-flow forecast. The difference between
the two is important. The *profits forecast* looks at how much the
partners earn from the day-to-day activities of running the practice,
usually over a 12-month period. It would take into account those
items of income and expenditure that have been earned or
incurred, but not yet received or paid, and would ignore expenses
on fixed assets and drawings, as there are not day-to-day expenses
of running the practice. In the case of fixed assets, the benefit of
the expense will be found for many years to come (not just the 12
months of the accounting period) and the drawings are in fact the
partners withdrawing their profits.

A profits forecast gives the GP the ability to see objectively
whether his or her practice is achieving below or above average
profitability. There are a number of independent publications
showing the average source of income to be achieved by GPs and
the forecast will enable a critical appraisal of the practice's results.
Some GPs will have a basic minimum earnings requirement, and
the GP will need to be certain that the practice can, in a 12-month
period, meet their requirements. If not, the GP may have to make
changes to the intended means of running the practice.

Having prepared a profits forecast, the GP should know with
some accuracy, the practice's profitability. This in turn needs to be
translated into another forecast, a *cash-flow forecast*. As stated
previously, the profits forecast is made up of items involved in the
day-to-day running of the practice and includes items when they are
earned or incurred. A cash-flow forecast looks at every source of
income or expense that is likely to pass through the practice bank
account (including fixed assets, drawings and partners' tax) and
includes items on the date the expense passes through the bank
account or when the income is received (Box 8.2).

Box 8.2
Forecasting types

1. Profits forecast (see Figure 8.1):
   – How much the partners earn from day to day. Identifies the core profitability of the practice.
2. Cash-flow forecast (see Figure 8.2):
   – All sources of income or expenses. Predicts the effect
   on the practice's solvency.

The difference between the two statements is fundamental.
Managing the cash flow is quite separate from establishing whether
the practice is profitable. Businesses that go into liquidation or
individuals who are made bankrupt do so, not because they are
unprofitable (many are in fact highly profitable), but because they
are unable to pay their debts on time.

Business plan 1995/96

Drs A, B, C and D

Profit (income and expenditure) forecast 1st October 1995 to 30th September 1996

	RATE	QTY	Q/E DEC 1995	QTY	Q/E MAR 1996	QTY	Q/E JUNE 1996	QTY	Q/E SEPT 1996	TOTAL
INCOME										
Allowances										
Basic practice allowance			6816		6816		6918		6918	27468
Seniority			660		660		670		670	2660
Postgraduate education allowance			2150		2150		2182		2182	8665
Capitation fees										
– Under 65	3.6500	6600	24090	6730	24565	6860	25415	6990	25896	99965
– 65–74	4.8250	440	2123	450	2171	460	2253	470	2302	8849
– Over 75	9.3250	390	3637	400	3730	410	3881	420	3975	15223
Registration fees	6.4500	200	1290	200	1290	200	1309	200	1309	5199
Child health surveillance	10.6000	92	966	95	998	96	1023	98	1044	4031
Target payments										
–Vaccinations, Age 2			2340		2340		2375		2375	9430
–Vaccinations, Age 5			515		515		523		523	2077
– Cytology			2401		2401		2437		2437	9676
Sessions payments										
Health promotion clinics										
– Band 3			2031		2072		2113		2154	8370
– Diabetes			360		360		360		360	1440
– Asthma			360		360		360		360	1440
Minor surgery	106.20	12	1274	12	1274	12	1294	12	1294	5136
Service fees										
Night visits			1100		1100		1117		1117	4433
Temporary residents										
– Up to 15 days	8.60	15	129	15	129	15	131	15	131	520
– Over 15 days	12.90	35	452	35	452	35	458	35	458	1820
Contraceptive services	3.40	900	3060	900	3060	900	3106	900	3106	12332
Emergency treatment	21.45	5	107	5	107	5	109	5	109	432
Immediately necessary treatment	8.60	5	43	5	43	5	44	5	44	173
Maternity medical services	90.99	50	4500	50	4500	50	4568	50	4568	18135

Figure 8.1

Profits forecast (continued on p. 166)

	RATE	QTY	Q/E DEC 1995	QTY	Q/E MAR 1996	QTY	Q/E JUNE 1996	QTY	Q/E SEPT 1996	TOTAL
Income (*continued*)										
Service fees (*continued*)										
Vaccinations										
– Tetanus	3.55	30	107	30	107	30	108	30	108	429
– Rubella	3.55	10	36	10	36	10	36	10	36	143
– 15-year-old boosters	3.55	10	36	10	36	10	36	10	36	143
– Travel	3.55	200	710	200	710	200	721	200	721	2 861
Reimbursements										
Rent			6 000		6 000		6 000		6 000	24 000
Rates and water rates			2 200		2 200		2 200		2 200	8 800
Staff costs										
– Salaries and NIC			25 200		25 200		25 200		25 200	100 800
– Trainee			7 500		7 500		7 500		7 500	30 000
– Training			0		0		0		0	0
Computer maintenance			500		500		508		508	2 015
Drugs and vaccinations			2 002		1 752		1 503		1 503	6 760
Other fees										
Private fees			1 200		1 200		1 200		1 200	4 800
Teaching			150		150		150		150	600
Training grant			1 168		1 169		1 169		1 169	4 675
Bank deposit interest			300		300		300		300	1 200
Fundholding/management allowance			4 375		4 375		8 750		8 750	26 250
TOTAL INCOME			111 887		112 326		118 025		118 712	460 950

EXPENDITURE

Staff salaries and welfare	35 000	35 000	35 000	35 000	140 000
Trainee	7 500	7 500	7 500	7 500	30 000
Locum	3 000	3 000	3 000	3 000	12 000
Relief services	2 500	2 500	2 500	2 500	10 000
Drugs and instruments	2 000	1 475	1 475	1 475	6 425
Rates and water rates	2 200	2 200	2 200	2 200	8 800
Light and heat	800	800	800	800	3 200
Insurance	350	350	350	350	1 400
Repairs and maintenance	350	350	350	350	1 400
Computer maintenance	1 000	1 000	1 000	1 000	4 000
Lease of equipment	400	400	400	400	1 600
Printing, postage and stationery	2 000	2 000	2 000	2 000	8 000
Telephone	1 200	1 200	1 200	1 200	4 800
Books and journals	50	50	50	50	200
Professional subscriptions	50	50	50	50	200
Cleaning and laundry	1 400	1 400	1 400	1 400	5 600
General expenses	600	600	600	600	2 400
Fundholding expenditure	4 375	4 375	8 750	8 750	26 250
NHS levies	250	250	250	250	1 000
Accountancy	800	800	800	800	3 200
Legal fees	500	500	500	500	2 000
Bank interest and charges	100	100	100	100	400
Loan interest	5 000	5 000	5 000	5 000	20 000
TOTAL EXPENDITURE	71 425	70 900	75 275	75 275	292 875
NET PROFIT	40 462	41 426	42 750	43 437	168 075

Figure 8.1 (*continued*)

Business plan 1995/96

Drs A, B, C and D

Cashflow forecast – 1st October 1995 to 30th September 1996

INCOME	OCT	NOV	DEC	JAN	FEB	MAR	APRIL	MAY	JUNE	JULY	AUG	SEPT	TOTAL
Fees and allowances	5300	5300	50692	5300	5300	50692	5300	5300	51380	5300	5300	52945	248109
Less: superannuation	0	0	-2500	0	0	-2500	0	0	-2500	0	0	-2500	-10000
Reimbursements													
Rent	1340	1340	3320	1340	1340	3320	1340	1340	3320	1340	1340	3320	24000
Rates and water rates	733	733	733	733	733	733	733	733	733	733	733	733	8800
Staff costs													
– Salaries and NIC	4000	4000	17200	4000	4000	17200	4000	4000	17200	4000	4000	17200	100800
– Trainee	1000	1000	5500	1000	1000	5500	1000	1000	5500	1000	1000	5500	30000
– Training	0	0	0	0	0	0	0	0	0	0	0	0	0
Courses and conferences	0	0	0	0	0	0	0	0	0	0	0	0	0
Computer maintenance	0	0	500	0	0	500	0	0	508	0	0	508	2015
Drugs and vaccinations	498	498	1006	756	498	498	501	501	501	501	501	501	6760
Other fees													
Private fees	400	400	400	400	400	400	400	400	400	400	400	400	4800
Teaching	50	50	50	50	50	50	50	50	50	50	50	50	600
Training grant	0	0	1168	0	0	1169	0	0	1169	0	0	1169	4675
Bank deposit interest	100	100	100	100	100	100	100	100	100	100	100	100	1200
Fundholding/management allowance	1458	1458	1458	1458	1458	1458	2917	2917	2917	2917	2917	2917	26250
TOTAL INCOME	14880	14880	79628	15138	14880	79121	16341	16341	81278	16341	16341	82843	448009
EXPENDITURE													
Practice expenditure	23808	23808	28808	23633	23633	23633	25092	25092	25092	25092	25092	25092	292875
Doctors' drawings	10000	10000	10000	10000	10000	10000	10000	10000	10000	10000	10000	10000	120000
Doctors' taxation	0	0	0	15000	0	0	0	0	0	15000	0	0	30000
Capital purchases	0	0	0	0	0	0	0	0	0	0	0	0	0
Repayment of loan capital	0	0	2000	0	0	2000	0	0	2000	0	0	2000	8000
TOTAL EXPENDITURE	33808	33808	35808	48633	33633	35633	35092	35092	37092	50092	35092	37092	450875
SURPLUS BROUGHT FORWARD	25000	6071	-12857	30962	-2534	-21287	22200	3449	-15302	28885	-4866	-23617	25000
SURPLUS/DEFICIT FOR THE MONTH	-18929	-18929	43819	-33496	-18754	43487	-18751	-18751	44186	-33751	-18751	45751	-2866
SURPLUS CARRIED FORWARD	6071	-12857	30962	-2534	-21287	22200	3449	-15302	28885	-4866	-23617	22134	22134

Figure 8.2
Cash-flow forecast

Interested outside
parties

The two outside parties likely to be most difficult with financial problems are the practice's bankers and the Inland Revenue. The bankers are obviously going to have their own view of the practice's cash flow. They will see it on a day-to-day basis. The cash flow may vary substantially over the year with troughs every 2 months and peaks when the health authority pay the quarter-end fees due. If the bankers can be shown in advance both the likely profitability of the practice and the management of the cash flow with which they can see future peaks, they will be able to be supportive to the practice in financing those troughs. They will, of course, want to be remunerated, but will be prepared to reduce their charges where their needs are explained in advance of being required. The Inland Revenue require the partners' tax to be paid twice a year. A cash-flow forecast should enable the practice to ensure that a sufficient level of profits are available to discharge the tax liability. In practical terms, many practices set up a separate tax account in a building society or bank deposit account to collect on a monthly basis a sixth of the half-year's tax. The practice accountant should be able to advise in advance the likely tax liability and this rather enforced method of saving for tax, should avoid any problems with the Inland Revenue. The joint and several liability between partners for partnership tax will be withdrawn shortly, but many practices will continue to put aside each partner's personal tax liability in a tax account.

Drawings
prediction

The completion of the cash-flow forecast will enable the partners to see what funds are available for them to draw each month. To maximize the efficiency of the practice's cash flow, the partners may choose to take out only those funds which are available. This may mean that for some months of the year, especially those months where the practice's tax is payable, there are no funds to be allocated to partner's drawings. The alternative is to pay a regular fixed drawing each month. This should be possible having prepared the profits forecast and the cash-flow forecast but, in view of the bank facilities required in those months of heavy expenditure, the support of the bank must be obtained in advance of those facilities being required.

Conclusion

It is not simply enough to prepare the profits forecast and cash-flow forecast, and then consign them to a drawer never to be seen again. As mentioned previously, the forecasts are a prediction of likely events and need to be updated on a regular basis as events unfold. A monthly review should be adequate. In addition, there may be pointers during the year that would lead the GP to question the validity of the forecasts. A reconciled bank balance moving steadily into debt at a rate greater than predicted in the cash-flow forecast should prompt an urgent reappraisal of the forecasts.

To summarize, the profits forecast identifies the core profitability of the practice. The cash-flow forecast predicts the effect on the practice's solvency, i.e. whether the funds required will be available.

PURPOSE OF ANNUAL ACCOUNTS – INDIVIDUAL COMPONENTS
The annual accounts, as the name suggests, cover a period of 12 months. To many GPs, the main purpose was to provide the Inland Revenue with sufficient information to issue an agreed income tax assessment, but this misses the point of the accounts. The accounts provide an objective historical record of the financial performance of the practice and, provided they are prepared promptly, will be a useful tool in making financial decisions. Three months after the year end is an ideal time period to have the accounts completed. The purpose of the accounts is to assess the normal profitability of the practice.

Fundamental components of the accounts
The accounts themselves comprise two pages, the profit and loss account (sometimes known as the income and expenditure account) and the balance sheet. All other pages and information

Box 8.3
Fundamental components of the accounts

> 1. Profit and loss account:
>   – Covers a time period and compares the day-to-day income and expenditure.
> 2. Balance sheet:
>   – Shows the assets and liabilities of the practice on the last day of the accounting period.

are subordinate to these pages (Box 8.3). A sample set of practice accounts are shown in the Appendix.

Profit and loss account

The profit and loss account covers a time period (normally 12 months) and compares the day-to-day income of a practising GP to the day-to-day expenses. Significant one-off payments for items such as purchasing fixtures and fittings, computers and premises are excluded, as these are not expenses incurred on a day-to-day basis. Significant one-off receipts, such as an improvement grant, would also be excluded. The *purpose* is to be able to ascertain the normal profitability of a practice, and the inclusion of non-routine expenses or income would distort the message. By reviewing the profits of a practice, the GP would be able to see how they compare to the average practice, how they compare to his or her own previous performance and, if they have the services of a specialist accountant, how they compare towards his or her own potential.

Balance sheet

The balance sheet is the other main page in the accounts. Unlike the profit and loss account, which covers an accounting period, this page shows the assets and liabilities of the practice on the last day of the accounting period. Assets are split between fixed and current. Fixed assets are those that, in simple terms, will have an enduring lifespan of more than 12 months. These include fixtures and fittings, computers, premises, etc. Current assets include those assets that will be turned to cash in the next 12 months, e.g. stocks of drugs, debtors, and bank funds and cash themselves. Deducted from these are the practice's liabilities, the amounts they owe to suppliers, to the Inland Revenue, for repayment of loans, etc. The net difference between the assets and the liabilities is the value or wealth of the practice.

The ownership of the practice is shown in the capital accounts (sometimes known as current accounts). Each partner's share of the wealth is shown in his or her own individual capital account. Apart from the introduction of an individual's own funds or an exceptional withdrawal, a GP's wealth (and therefore the practice's) is enhanced by drawing less profits than are being earned. Conversely, a GP's wealth (and, therefore, the practice's) is diminished by drawing more profits than are being earned. It

Case example 1
Scene setting

For example, Drs Smith and Jones share profits equally. Profits are currently £100 000. Dr Smith pays superannuation including added years of £4000 while Dr Jones pays superannuation of £2000. Dr Smith has high personal expenses, the result of which is that his tax liability paid through the practice, is only £3500. Dr Jones has extensive outside income, the result of which is that his tax liability, paid through the practice, is £9000. What should their monthly drawings be?

	Total	Dr Smith	Dr Jones
Share of profits	£100 000	£50 000	£50 000
Less:			
Superannuation	£6 000	£4 000	£2 000
Income tax	£12 500	£3 500	£9 000
Net annual drawings	£81 500	£42 500	£39 000
Monthly drawings	£6 791	£3 541	£3 250

is important to appreciate that drawings do not include simply the cash or cheques taken each month but also, an individual's superannuation contributions, added years and additional voluntary contributions (AVCs) and, where the practice collects the partnership's tax liability, each partner's share of that liability. Two partners sharing profits equally may well have different superannuation payments, owing to one partner buying added years, and will almost certainly have differing tax liabilities. This would mean in practice that they should take differing amounts of monthly drawings to ensure that, at the end of the year, their respective shares of the wealth are equal.

If the partners had taken equal drawings then, once the income tax payments and superannuation contributions had been made, they would have different balances on their respective current accounts. This would, in fact, mean that the two equal partners would have differing financial commitments to the practice, which would be quite wrong.

It fairly common to see accounts with such differing balances, usually a result of poor financial advice. The situation should not be ignored, as the balances do translate to cash as and when a partner leaves, retires or dies.

Valuation of assets It was mentioned above that part of the wealth of the practice was reflected by the fixed assets. How these are valued in the accounts will have a direct impact on the value of the practice and, therefore, the partners' capital accounts. The accountants will reduce the value of the assets each year over the life of the asset, a process known as depreciation. This will be arbitrary, and is not intended to reflect the possible sale price of the asset. Assets such as computer equipment purchased with the assistance of grants, or assets purchased with fundholding savings will be shown at net cost in the accounts, and this is the figure used to calculate depreciation. The asset may, of course, be sold at a value closer to the gross cost. Surgery premises will undoubtedly cost more than they are worth on the open market. Negative equity will be apparent in many cases. If, however, the premises are valued in terms of the level of reimbursement received by the practice (which is likely to be much more than the open market), the negative equity should disappear. These points illustrate the number of various options in terms of asset valuation and, therefore, how easily the value of a partner's capital account can be affected. In order to avoid conflict at a time when these figures are calculated, it is suggested that the practice specifically refer to the valuation method in the practice agreement.

Additional useful information The annual accounts should be used as a management tool. As such, they should be up to date and, also, include further information such as analysis of the General Medical Services (GMS) income, comparative figures for the previous year, breakdown of reimbursements, summary of other income and a per-patient breakdown of the items of service.

SOURCES OF INCOME AND EXPENDITURE – DETAILED COMPONENTS

The new contract of 1990 set out the manner in which GPs are to be remunerated. It introduced for the first time the concept of targets, and removed a number of fee items which had simple criteria to meet. For example, group practice allowance became payable where three GPs work together. Vocational training allowance became payable annually provided the GP is vocationally trained. The new contract seeks to ensure that GPs receive an average remuneration, which, provided they have an average list size, they should be able to do. An average list size is currently 1887 patients.

Income refers to the income generated by the GP in the normal practising capacity. It includes all GMSC sources of income, reimbursements, outside commitments and private income. It is matched by practice expenditure in achieving that income, such as staff costs, premises costs, administration costs and financial costs, but does not include significant expenditure on assets that will have a life in excess of the current accounting period. This expenditure is referred to as fixed assets.

The individual sources of income are given below.

PRACTICE INCOME

Non-items of service payment

Capitation fees

The health authority will make a payment to the GP for every patient on the GP's list. The payment is made quarterly at three rates, depending on the age of the patient. The rates are:

- ◆ Under 65 years   £16.05 per annum
- ◆ Between 65 and 74 years   £21.20 per annum
- ◆ Age 75 and over   £41.00 per annum

The average practice has an age distribution of which 89% of the patients are less than 65 years, 6% of the patients are age 65–74, and 5% are age 75 and over. It is a common factor for practices to have more patients on their list than actually exist. This occurs predominantly in inner-city areas with high patient turnover rates. These 'ghosts' can account for 30% of a list and, whilst attractive from a capitation point of view, can be expensive in failing to meet targets (see later). The introduction of a direct computerized link between the health authority and the practice (GP links) will in time remove all 'ghosts'. A practice seeking to take on a vacant list may have to take steps to see how many of the potential patients are in fact 'ghosts'.

Basic practice allowance

The basic practice allowance (BPA) is payable to a GP principal, either a sole practitioner or a partner. The full BPA is payable to a full-time practitioner (available at least 26 hours per week) who has either 1200 or more patients on their list, or the average list of the partnership is 1200 or more patients per partner. The full annual BPA is £7488. A reduced payment is made for a smaller list size, starting at 400 patients and increasing in stages up to 1200 patients.

A half-time practitioner (available at least 13 hours per week) can claim a BPA up to a maximum of 600 patients (currently £4680) and a three-quarter time practitioner (available at least 18 hours per week) can claim up to a maximum of 900 patients (currently £6400).

It is curious that a half-time practitioner is entitled to 62.5% of the full BPA while a three-quarter time practitioner is entitled to 85.42% of the full BPA. This is a factor often overlooked when a practice is planning to recruit new partners and determine the needs, costs and benefits.

Leave payment

Leave pay is in effect an interest-free loan from the health authority to the GP. It is given in the quarter ending 30 June and recovered quarterly during the rest of the year, ending on the following 31 March. The amount of the leave payment is restricted to 20% of the appropriate basic practice allowance. Applications for the payment must be made by 15 April.

Seniority

This allowance is paid for a GP who has satisfied two time-based criteria: the number of years as a registered doctor with the GMC, and the number of years as an NHS GP principal. Some GPs keep this allowance themselves, while others share the income in the partnership pool. Both methods are acceptable but, whichever basis is adopted, should be referred to in the partnership agreement. The levels of payments are as follows:

- Registered with the GMC for 11 years, working as a GP principal for 7 years   £465
- Registered with the GMC for 18 years, working as a GP principal for 14 years   £2425
- Registered with the GMC for 25 years, working as a GP principal for 21 years   £5235

Deprivation payments

The Jarman index is used to define areas of the country that are deemed to be deprived. A deprivation payment is made for each patient on the GP's list residing in a deprived area. The purpose of the payments is to compensate those practices who are unable to maximize their targets and other variable sources of income, due to the difficult nature of their patients or location. The areas are selected on information taken from the latest census, with changes last effected in June 1995 based on the 1991 census. The current rates of payment are:

◆ Patients in a high-level deprived area   £11.20 per annum
◆ Patients in medium-level deprived area   £8.40 per annum
◆ Patients in a low-level deprived area   £6.45 per annum

The criteria for the health authority making such a payment is the patient's postcode. Therefore, it is vital to ensure that the patients' postcodes are correctly recorded by the health authority.

Rural practice payments

This scheme provides for payment from a Rural Practices Fund. A single-handed GP is eligible to be credited with Rural Practice Units if 20% of the patients live at least 3 miles from the main surgery. For a partnership, the calculations are made on the basis of the partnership list as a whole, not each partner's individual list.

If, having qualified for rural practice payments, the percentage falls below 20% but more than 19%, the health authority has the discretion to continue payment of the scheme for up to four more quarters. The calculation of units increases from one unit for distances of at least 3 miles but less than four miles, up to ten miles for distances of at least 7 but less than 10 miles, and two additional units for each additional mile or part of a mile.

There are also additional walking units for each part of the route that has to be walked, refunds of exceptional out-of-pocket expenses (e.g. ferry charges, toll charges, etc.), and special arrangements for lighthouses and islands.

The unit payment is 0.219p for 1996/97 with a proposed increase of 4.4% in the Rural Practice Fund.

Child health surveillance

In order to undertake and be paid for these services, the GP must be included on the health authority's child health surveillance list. A fee of £11.65 is paid for each child under 5 years of age for the provision of services set down by the health authority. The GP should check their list of eligible children to the health authority's list.

Minor surgery

In order to undertake these services, the GP must be included on the health authority's minor surgery list to claim a fee. The fee is payable to an approved GP for providing minor surgery to their patients or the patients of their partners. It is possible for one approved GP to undertake all the minor surgery work for the partnership and to claim fees on behalf of the other partners.

The maximum claim is three sessional payments per GP per quarter. Each session consists of five surgical procedures which include aspirations, injections, incisions, excisions, currete cautery and cryocautery, and the removal of foreign bodies.

The sessional payment is £116.80, i.e. the fee for five procedures. The maximum claim is three sessions per quarter, therefore, the maximum fee per GP is £1401.60. This fee is not reduced for part-time GPs.

Registration fees

A fee is payable for a medical examination of a new patient if the examination is conducted within 3 months of admitting the patient on to the GP's list. The health authority has the discretion to extend the 3-month time period for up to 2 years. The fee payable is £7.10 per registration check.

Registration fees can also be claimed where a partner leaves, and that partner's patients are reregistered on another partner's list. No fee is payable for children under 5 or where the patient had such an examination within the practice in the last 12 months.

Health promotion clinics

If a practitioner participates in a health promotion programme, he or she will be eligible for payment from the Health Promotion and the Chronic Disease Management (CDM) Fund. The health promotion programme remunerates the GP according to which band the programme is in. The payment level is set on the basis of a national average list size and is, therefore, adjusted to the list size of the practice. GPs are paid a flat-rate payment for the CDM programme, irrespective of list size. CDM payments are available for either a diabetes CDM programme, an asthma CDM programme, or both. GPs in partnership can carry out joint programmes.

Each health promotion or CDM programme must receive prior approval from the health authority.

The current fee levels are:

- Band 1 per 1884 patients   £450
- Band 2 per 1884 patients   £1220
- Band 3 per 1884 patients   £2260
- Asthma clinics   £395
- Diabetes clinics   £395

Health promotion clinics represent the influence and philosophy behind the new contract, perhaps more than anything else. The original payment structure of £45 per clinic allowed some GPs to earn far more than the Department of Health expected (it also showed the resourcefulness of some GPs) and so the scheme was changed to reward those GPs carrying a greater programme of health promotion than others. Unfortunately, and somewhat surprisingly, 83% of all practices are in band 3, which dilutes the payment to be made from the fund and enhances the downwards trend in GPs available earnings.

Cervical cytology targets

A GP will receive a target payment at the higher rate if, on the first day of a given quarter, at least 80% of the eligible women on the GP's list aged between 25 and 64 have had an adequate smear during a period 5 years and 6 months preceding the claim. A lower rate payment will be made if at least 50% of the eligible women have had an adequate smear. The targets are assessed over the partnership list size as a whole and not each partner's separate list.

The actual payment is based on the number of eligible patients, compared to the national average number of eligible patients for a practice. To reach the appropriate target, the test is whether the proportion of the list have been smeared, not whether those patients were smeared by the practice. The actual payment, however, is reduced by that proportion of the patients who were tested by outside organizations such as local authority clinics.

Women who have had hysterectomies are excluded from the target calculation.

The maximum higher target payment for an average number of patients is £2610. The maximum lower target payment for an average number of patients is £870.

Immunizations for children aged 2 years and under – targets

A GP will receive a target payment at the higher rate if, on the first day of a given quarter, at least 90% of the eligible children on the GP's list aged 2 or less have achieved full immunization. A lower rate payment will be made if at least 70% of the eligible children have achieved full immunization. The targets are assessed over the partnership list size as a whole and not each partner's separate list.

Similar to cytology smears, reaching the target depends on the number of eligible children who have achieved full immunization, the actual payment depends on the number of children immunized by the GP or their practice.

The maximum higher target payment for an average number of patients is £2340. The maximum lower target payment for an average number of patients is £780.

Immunizations for children aged 5 years and under – targets

A GP will receive a target payment at the higher rate if, on the first day of a given quarter, at least 90% of the eligible children on the GP's list aged 5 or less have had reinforcing doses of suggested immunizations. A lower rate payment will be made if at least 70% of the eligible children have had reinforcing doses of suggested immunizations. The targets are assessed over the partnership list size as a whole and not each partner's separate list.

Similar to cytology smears, reaching the target depends on the number of eligible children who have had reinforcing doses of suggested immunizations. The actual payment depends on the number of children immunized by the GP or their practice.

The maximum higher target payment for an average number of patients is £690. The maximum lower target payment for an average number of patients is £230.

The concept of targets is another reason for the continued pressure on GP's profits towards the average. Far more practices reach the targets now than when the new contract was first introduced, with the result that the pool is more evenly spread. Whether it is still appropriate to use a targeting system is open to question.

Postgraduate education allowance (PGEA)

A GP will be paid an allowance if he or she has attended 25 days of accredited postgraduate education spread over the previous 5 years and has, during that time, attended at least two accredited courses in health promotion, disease management and service management.

A doctor becoming a GP more than 12 months after completing vocational training will be paid the full allowance where the first claim is made within 12 months and each subsequent claim is made within 15 months of the previous claim. The first claim should confirm the GP has attended at least 5 days of accredited courses within the year. The second claim should confirm the GP has attended at least 10 days of accredited courses within the 2 years preceding the claim. The third claim should confirm the GP has attended at least 15 days of accredited courses within the 3 years preceding the claim. The fourth claim should confirm the GP has attended at least 20 days of accredited courses within the 4 years preceding the claim.

A doctor becoming a GP for the first time within 12 months of completing vocational training will be paid the full allowance provided the claim is made within 12 months of completing vocational training. A reduced allowance is payable if the GP is unable to maintain the 5 year programme. The current full allowance is £2360.

Items of service payment

Maternity medical fees

A fee is paid for providing maternity services to patients. A GP who is not on the obstetric list providing these services, receives a lower level of fees for these services. In addition, an obstetrically approved GP can provide those services to women not on the GPs list of patients.

The antenatal care fee payable is dependent on the date a woman signs the acceptance application on form FP24. A miscarriage fee is payable if a woman's pregnancy ends before the 28th week and does not result in a live birth. Confinement care fees are payable where maternity medical services are provided during a confinement.

A GP providing maternity medical services to mother and child throughout the 14 days after confinement and carries out a full postnatal examination at or about 6 weeks after confinement, is paid the full fee. A partial fee is payable for each attendance during the 14 days after birth, up to a maximum of five such visits. A separate fee is payable for a full postnatal examination, at or about 6 weeks after birth.

The complete medical maternity services fee is paid to a GP who provides complete care during pregnancy, confinement and the postnatal period, and carries out the full postnatal examination at or about 6 weeks after birth.

The level of fees for GPs who are/are not on the obstetric list are as follows:

- ◆ Complete services   £186 /£107
- ◆ Antenatal care woman signing up to 16 weeks £100   /£58.55
- ◆ Antenatal care woman signing between 17 and 30 weeks   £73.35/£43.95
- ◆ Antenatal care woman signing up to 31 weeks and after   £50.20/£29.30
- ◆ Miscarriage fee   £62   /£38.70
- ◆ Confinement care   £42.85/£24.80
- ◆ Complete postnatal care   £42.85/£30.30
- ◆ Partial care attendance
  - – Each attendance   £5.69 /£4.05
  - – Maximum   £28.50/£20.10
- ◆ Full postnatal examination   £14.25/£10.20

Contraceptive services

There are two types of fees payable for providing contraceptive services: the ordinary fee when a GP gives advice and conducts any necessary examination, and an intrauterine device fee (IUD) when a GP fits an IUD and provides care for a period of 12 months. The annual ordinary fee for providing contraceptive advice is £14.90 while the IUD fee is £49.80.

Night visits and out of hours

This item has attracted more political debate than any other in recent times. It is cited as one of the core reasons for poor recruitment and led to the setting up of groups of GPs working in cooperatives, with the Department of Health setting aside a fund of £45 million.

GPs can bid for a share of the out-of-hours fund and every bid must be cost effective and maintain or improve standards of care for patients out of surgery hours. The bid can apply for funding to cover premises, staffing and equipment.

The payment for night visits was changed on 1 January 1996. Each GP receives a flat rate payment of £2165 plus £21.65 for each face to face consultation between 10 p.m. and 8 a.m. The fee can be generated by any GP principal or doctor eligible to be a principal, and by GP registrars, assistants, locums and associates.

GPs now have the ability to transfer responsibility for out-of-hours care to another GP, and must come to a private financial arrangement to do so. The hours that can be transferred are from 7 p.m. to 8 a.m. weekdays, and 1 p.m. Saturdays to 8 a.m. Mondays.

Temporary residents

If a GP actually treats a person temporarily resident in the area for more than 24 hours and less than 3 months, the GP can claim a temporary resident's fee. A lower fee is paid if the temporary resident expects to remain in the area for less than 15 days from first treatment, with a higher fee payable if the temporary resident expects to be in the area for more than 15 days. The lower fee is £9.45. The higher fee is £14.20.

Where the only treatment provided attracts an item of service fee for vaccinations, immunizations, contraceptive services, maternity medical services or the arrest of a dental haemorrhage, only that fee can be claimed and not the item of service fee.

GPs cannot take on patients in the area on a temporary basis if the patients are permanently resident in the area.

Emergency treatment fee

A GP can claim an emergency treatment fee for providing a service in an accident or emergency to a person not registered with the practice and whose total length of stay in the area is for less than 24 hours.

If the service was provided to a patient of a neighbouring practice, the health authority may deduct the payment from the patient's own GP, if that GP was not available to provide the service personally. This does not apply between the hours of 10 p.m. and 8 a.m. The fee is £23.60.

Immediate necessary treatment

If a person applies for treatment and the GP is unwilling to accept the patient or to treat the person as a temporary resident, but the patient requires treatment, the GP is obliged to supply all immediate necessary treatment.

The immediate necessary treatment fee is:

- Where the patient is resident in the area for less
  than 15 days   £9.45
- Where the patient is resident in the area for more
  than 15 days   £14.20

Arrest of dental haemorrhage

A GP who arrests a dental haemorrhage in a patient can claim a fee. The higher fee is payable for attendance while the lower fee relates to the removal of dental plugs and/or stitches.

- The lower fee is   £16.10
- The higher fee is   £23.60

Service of an anaesthetist

A fee is payable when the services of a second doctor are required for the administration of a general anaesthetic (except in the case of the provision of maternity services). The fee is payable when the anaesthetic is administered by the GP responsible for the patient or by the second doctor. The fee is not payable if the anaesthetic is given under arrangements made by the hospital services. The fee for this service is £39.95.

Vaccinations and immunizations

A GP vaccinating a patient in accordance with public policy is able to claim a fee for the service. The patient must be either on the GP's list, a temporary resident or staying in the area for less than 24 hours. The vaccinations included in this section are travel immunizations, tetanus, anthrax, rabies, infectious hepatitis, etc. The fees for higher rate items are £5.65. The fees for lower rate items are £3.90.

Reimbursements It is a principle under the new contract that GPs are reimbursed for some of their expenses to a great extent. Since the 1990 New Contract, the levels of reimbursements have been challenged and put under greater pressure than at any other time. It should be appreciated that any downward trend in GP's reimbursements will inevitably lead to downward pressure on GP's profits. The main reimbursements are as follows.

Rent and rates

The GP will be eligible for rent and rate reimbursements if they have at least 100 patients. The scheme is designed to cover the cost to the GP of providing accommodation either rented or owned by the GP. If the GP rents the premises, provided the health authority is satisfied with the level of accommodation provided, it will reimburse all the rent, rates, water rates and refuse charges. If the GP owns the premises, he or she will either be reimbursed on a cost rent basis or a notional rent basis. Cost rent seeks to reimburse the interest charges on the cost of a new or modified surgery. It should be noted that the repayment of capital is up to the GP. The calculations are complicated and, before the GPs commit themselves to anything, they should ask the health authority for the interim cost rent, which will give them a good indication of the likely reimbursement. The GPs will also have to consider whether they wish to be reimbursed on a fixed or variable rate basis, which will depend on whether they have a fixed or variable rate loan. One important point which is often forgotten is that the fixed rate of reimbursement is the rate prevailing at the date the GPs sign the building tenders, not the date the loan is agreed. The dates of signing the tender and agreeing the loan should be as close as possible.

An alternative to cost rent is for the GP to be reimbursed under notional rent. This is assessed every 3 years by the district valuer (part of the Inland Revenue) who determines the current market rent that might reasonably be expected to be paid for the premises. If a GP is on cost rent, he or she has the option every 3 years to switch to notional rent, but the switch cannot be in the opposite direction. The GP owner-occupier will also be reimbursed for rates, water rates and refuse collection.

If the GP undertakes private work at, or associated with the surgery, the reimbursements will be abated if the private work exceeds 10% of total income.

Staff reimbursements

Before 1990, each full-time GP was reimbursed 70% of the cost of two full-time equivalent members of staff and 100% of the employers National Insurance Contributions (NIC). This radically changed in the new contract, where the levels of reimbursement are at the health authority's discretion. In many cases, this works in the GP's favour, with some staff members reimbursed at 100%. There are trends to reduce the reimbursement and some health authorities in particular are less generous than others. The goal should still be 70%, but as sickness and overtime are rarely reimbursed, GPs are having to accept a lower rate of reimbursement unless in many cases they change their employee contracts.

Fundholders are in the position of being able to negotiate a budget for their staff costs, which gives them, theoretically, a greater degree of freedom and flexibility.

Other reimbursements

There are also reimbursements available for:

♦ Locums, owing to sickness.
♦ GP maternity leave.
♦ Computer expenses.

- The doctors retainer scheme.
- Courses and training.
- Improvements.
- Trainee.
- Assistants allowance.

PRACTICE
EXPENDITURE

GP practices are businesses and have to pay expenses out of income. In order for a practice to be profitable, it must not only maximize the income of the practice, but also control the expenditure. The expenses of general practice can be divided into two categories: those incurred by the practice as business expenses, and those incurred personally as business expenses. The Inland Revenue do not draw any distinction between the two categories of expenses.

Typical expenses incurred personally would be:

- Motor expenses (usually proportions of two cars).
- Professional subscriptions.
- Telephone and mobile telephone (proportions of both).
- Personally bought drugs and instruments.
- Dry cleaning and laundry.
- Personal security.
- Professional proportion of use of home.
- Printing, postage and stationery.
- Personal accountancy.
- Medical books and journals.
- Staff wages (spouse or nanny).
- Staff pension scheme (for spouse).
- General expenses.

Typical expenses incurred by the practice are shown in the attached sample of accounts (Appendix). A method of assessing the control and level of expenses is shown in a later section.

TAXATION OF THE
PARTNERSHIP

At the time of writing, the UK taxation system is in the process of change. The preceding year basis of taxation is being replaced by the current year basis and the historical assessment by the Inland Revenue of a practice's tax liability is being replaced with the practice assessing themselves (Box 8.4). The effect of these changes will be to put a greater responsibility on the practice to

Box 8.4
Taxation changes

	Old	New
Basis of taxation	Preceding year	Current year
Tax liability assessment	Inland Revenue	Practice

deal promptly with their tax affairs, with particular responsibility on the senior partner in a practice and a new penalty regime for non-compliance.

Preceding year of assessment

1995/96 is the last year of the preceding year basis. The accounting year this relates to depends on the practice's year end. The principle of the preceding year basis is that the practice's profits for an accounting year are taxed in the next complete fiscal (6 April to 6 April) year. For example, a practice with a year end of 31 March 1995 will be taxed in 1995/96 (the next complete fiscal year is 6 April 1995 to 5 April 1996). A practice with a year end of 30 June 1994 will be taxed in 1995/96 (the next complete fiscal year is 6 April 1995 to 5 April 1996). From this example, it is clear that a June year end is preferable as the delay between the date the profits are earned and the date the tax is paid is 10 months more than it would be with a March year end. Because of this factor, many practices have a 30 June year end as it is the earliest year end coinciding with a quarter end when the health authority send the balance of fees and allowances earned.

The current year basis

The current year basis replaces the preceding year basis and is introduced in 1997/98. The principle of the current year basis is that the profits are taxed in the fiscal year in which the practice's accounting year ends. For example, an accounting year ended 30 June 1998 will be taxed in 1998/99 as will an accounting year end 31 March 1999 will be taxed in 1998/99. Once again, there is a difference in timing between earning the profits and paying the tax.

1996/97 – the transitional year

From the above explanation, 1995/96 is the last year of the preceding year basis while 1997/98 is the first year of the current year basis. This is one tax (fiscal) year missing, 1996/97. There are also two accounting years that have not been considered, e.g. June year end:

- Year ended 30/6/94   Taxed on preceding year basis   1995/96
- Year ended 30/6/95   ?
- Year ended 30/6/96   ?
- Year ended 30/6/97   Taxed on current year basis   1997/98

In order to calculate the profits taxable in the missing tax year 1996/97, the profits for the two years ended in the transitional year (in this case 30 June 1995 and 30 June 1996) are averaged to be left with the profits for an equivalent 12-month period.

The assessment and collection of tax

Until the year ended 5 April 1996, 1995/96 income tax was collected after the Inland Revenue received an individual's personal tax return, the practice accounts, partner's personal expenses and a computation showing how the profits should be shared between the partners. After the Inland Revenue have reviewed the information, the Inspector of Taxes agrees or questions this, and issues an assessment to collect the tax. Under this regime, the Inland Revenue can only investigate a taxpayer after making a discovery.

The Inland Revenue introduced self-assessment with effect 1996/97. As the title suggests, this is very different from the procedures mentioned above. In its place, each taxpayer has to complete a detailed tax return which calculates his or her individual tax liability. Each partnership completes a return from which each partner takes their own profit share and includes it on their own return. In principle, the individual pays his or her own tax liability when submitting the tax return with no submission of accounts. This procedure dispenses with the need for routine assessments, as a far greater responsibility is now placed on the taxpayer. To ensure compliance with the new regulations, the Inspectors of Taxes will be able to investigate taxpayers without the need to justify their actions.

It is possible to insure against the costs of an Inland Revenue investigation but, in the past, some taxpayers have taken the view that, with a reputable firm of accountants and a good history of acceptance of accounts without question, such insurance is unnecessary. This attitude needs to be looked at again. The Inland Revenue will, under self-assessment, investigate taxpayers affairs randomly. Even if the Inland Revenue are unable to find any mistakes or errors, the accountant's costs of defending the taxpayer will need to be paid and are likely to be substantial.

Allowable expenses

Tax-deductible expenses derive from antiquated tax law and the history of tax cases. The rules in practice are very different for the self-employed and the employed. The self-employed (most GPs fall into this category) have to justify that their expenses are 'wholly and exclusively incurred in the performance of their duties'. The employed have to justify that their expenses are 'wholly and exclusively *and necessarily* incurred in the performance of their duties'. The additional criteria of necessity makes a dramatic difference. The typical allowable expenses for the employed GP would be:

◆ Professional subscriptions.
◆ Some travelling and courses.

Most other expenses would be at the discretion of the Inland Revenue.

The typical allowance expenses for the self-employed GP are as mentioned above. As can be appreciated, the tax liability of the self-employed is considerably less than the employed.

National insurance contributions (NIC)

Self-employed GPs are obliged to pay both Class 2 and Class 4. Class 2 NIC is currently £6.05 per week irrespective of income. Class 4 NIC is for 1995/96 calculated at 6% of profit share in excess of £6860, up to a maximum profit share of £23 660. The maximum Class 4 NIC liability is, therefore, £1008.

Employed GPs (assuming they are in the NHS superannuation scheme) pay Class 1 NIC, which is 2% of the first £61 per week and 8.2% up to £455 per week. The maximum NIC paid by the employed GP would be £1689.16. In addition, the employer has to pay 10.2% on the first £61 and 7.2% on the balance with no upper limit.

Capital allowances

The cost of practice assets such as personal motor cars, computers, desks, etc. qualify for tax relief not as an expense, but as a capital allowance, claimed as a proportion of the cost each year. The allowance is given at the rate of 25% on the reduced balance brought forward (in tax terms called the written-down value brought forward – WDV b/f). For motor cars, the maximum eligible cost is £12 000. If the cost is in excess of £12 000, the allowance is restricted and calculated on the basis that WDV b/f is £12 000 (Box 8.5) e.g. car cost £15 000, computer costs £20 000.

Box 8.5
Capital allowances

	Motor car	Computer
Year 1:		
– Cost	£15 000	£20 000
– Capital allowance (restricted for car)	£3 000	£5 000
– Written-down value carried forward	£12 000	£15 000
Year 2:		
– Written down value brought forward	£12 000	£15 000
– Capital allowance @ 25%	£3 000	£3 750
– Written down value carried forward	£9 000	£11 250
Year 3:		
– Written down value brought forward	£9 000	£11 250
– Capital allowance @ 25%	£2 250	£2 813
– Written down value carried forward	£6 750	£8 437
Etc.		

FINANCIAL MONITORING AND METHODS OF MONITORING

Accountants use ratio analysis in reviewing the profitability and liquidity of clients and for investment purposes. General practice is, however, a unique business and most of the ratios generally used by accountants will be inappropriate. Accounting is not a science but an art, and any conclusions drawn have to be carefully considered to see if they are relevant.

Expenses ratios

The four key ratios dealing with expenses deal with staff costs, administrative expenses, financial and professional costs, and clinical assistance (outside medical help). All these ratios are shown as a percentage of the general medical services (GMS) income of the practice.

1. Staff efficiency ratio

The staff costs/GMS income ratio ignores staff reimbursements and looks at how efficiently the practice utilizes its staff. The ratio to aim for is 45–50% and, in general, the lower the better. If the practice is dispensing or has a nurse practitioner, a more subjective view should be taken. The relevance of this ratio is that many practices still employ staff on the basis of apparent need, rather than looking at whether this existing compliment of staff work efficiently. This itself is a hangover from the pre-1990 contract where, up to a maximum level, staff were automatically reimbursed at 70%.

2. Administration efficiency ratio

The administrative ratio/GMS income looks at how much the practice spends on the day-to-day running expenses. For this ratio, reimbursements are taken into account in reducing the expense. The ratio to aim for is between 8% and 13%.

3. Financial and professional ratio

The financial and professional costs/GMS income ratio would normally include the annual accountancy fees and any legal fees. On a year by year basis this should be about 2%.

4. Clinical assistance ratio

Finally, the clinical assistance/GMS income ratio looks at how much of the GMS income is spent on additional clinical help to the GPs. The net cost of an assistant, locum fees, deputizing fees and cooperative membership would be included. In some practices where the partners have the willingness and the numbers to cover each other, the percentage will be less than 1%. A single-handed GP cannot realistically aim for less than 10%, while a practice not wishing to do their own on call could spend up to 25% of their GMS income. This ratio is perhaps becoming the most useful in determining whether the practice is more profitable than another practice.

Income ratios   The income of the practice is split into two ratios. The fixed income per patient ratio and the effort-related income per patient ratio.

1. Fixed income per patient

The fixed income per patient ratio looks at the amount of income earned regardless of the efforts of the GP. This would include capitation fees, deprivation fees, basic practice allowances, PGEA and seniority. The fixed income per patient will depend on the location of the practice, and the age profile of the partners and the list size. Without deprivation, the fixed income per patient will be approximately £22.00 and, with average levels of deprivation, this increases to £26.00–£27.00.

2. Effort-related income per patient

The effort-related income per patient expresses all the other types of GMS income on a per patient basis. These would include items of service, targets, minor surgery, child health surveillance, etc. This is the ratio that can separate the low-earning GPs from the average or the high-earning GPs. The maximum that can normally be earned would be about £12.00 per patient. A figure of £10.00 or above should be regarded as high, while anything less should be examined to find the reason why.

3. Net profit per patient

Ultimately, the GP earns the net profit after all income and expenses have been taken into account. The average GP makes about £22.00 per patient in terms of profit, with some GPs able to increase this to £27.00–£28.00 and some unable to increase this beyond £15.00. Given that the average GP has some 2000 patients, the range of profitability for a GP is between £30 000 and £56 000 with few GPs falling outside this range.

4. Staff wages covered by reimbursement

Staff costs are reimbursed at the health authority's discretion. Just as the staff costs are the largest single expense, so the reimbursement must be critical to the practice's finances. It is always useful to check the level of reimbursement that the practice is receiving, especially now that neither sickness pay nor overtime are normally reimbursed.

These practice financial performance indicators are illustrated in the following example (Box 8.6).

These ratios can be applied to any practice and will give a direct indication and the specific reason to decide whether a practice is profitable. Comparing the ratios from one year to another will give the practice a trend on whether they are increasing or decreasing their efficiency. It is also useful to compare the ratios from one

Box 8.6
Practice financial performance indicators

Practice statistics for the year ending 31 March 1996

	1996	1995
Expenses ratios		
– Staff wages efficiency	$\frac{253\,323}{288\,433} = 87.83\%$	$\frac{221\,328}{307\,935} = 71.87\%$
– Administrative	$\frac{58\,026}{288\,433} = 20.12\%$	$\frac{35\,973}{307\,935} = 11.68\%$
– Financial and professional	$\frac{13\,239}{288\,433} = 4.59\%$	$\frac{4\,189}{307\,935} = 1.36\%$
– Clinical assistance	$\frac{75\,116}{288\,433} = 26.04\%$	$\frac{61\,575}{307\,935} = 19.99\%$
Income ratios		
– Income per patient	$\frac{288\,433}{9\,224} = £31.27$	$\frac{307\,935}{8\,947} = £34.42$
– Fixed income per patient	$\frac{177\,709}{9\,224} = £19.27$	$\frac{182\,879}{8\,947} = £20.44$
– Effort-related income per patient	$\frac{110\,724}{9\,224} = £12.00$	$\frac{125\,056}{8\,947} = £13.98$
– Net profit per patient	$\frac{149\,553}{9\,224} = £16.21$	$\frac{160\,513}{8\,947} = £17.94$
– Staff wages covered by reimbursement	$\frac{175\,012}{262\,495} = 66.67\%$	$\frac{146\,494}{218\,354} = 67.09\%$

practice to another, to see what is achievable, although in practice it will be difficult to obtain this information.

Where a practice has been encountering financial difficulties, it may wish to prepare accounts on a quarterly basis. Again, these same ratios will give a guide to the inherent trends within the practice.

The balance sheet, as explained above, illustrates the net asset value of the practice. Given that the practice may decrease its net assets by the partners overdrawing or increase its assets by underdrawing, the net assets should be compared to the figure in the previous year's accounts. If the figure remains constant, the inference will be that the partners are drawing equally to what they earn. If the figure is reducing, the inference will be that the partners are overdrawing, while an increasing figure will indicate the partners are underdrawing.

The above pointers will give the GP all the messages they need. Indeed, a bank manager recently commented to the writer that the ratio analysis in the accounts has enabled him to be more understanding and helpful to his GP customers.

FINANCIAL PLANNING AND DECISION-MAKING PRINCIPLES   The annual accounts provide the practice with a historical record of all that occurred in the previous accounting period. While this can be useful, it has a number of limitations in terms of future planning. In particular, it does not take into account changes within the practice and changes in the GP financial environment. For instance, the new fees for night visits will not be recorded in previous accounts, and a switch from a practice doing their own on call to joining a cooperative will have a profound effect on the practice finances.

Budgets/cash flows

The way to deal with this is to prepare a forecast of the profits for at least a year ahead. The forecast should only include those items that appear in the profit and loss account (i.e. it excludes partners' drawings, partners' tax, fixed assets), as the purpose of the forecast is to predict the long-term profitability of the practice. It would be helpful for the prediction to be made on a quarterly basis as this coincides with the dates GPs are paid. While this looks at the ongoing profitability of the practice, it does not predict whether the practice will have sufficient funds to meet its new objectives.

To deal with the funding requirements, a monthly cash-flow forecast should be prepared, predicting every item that is likely to pass through the practice's bank account. The forecast will indicate the time periods when any overdraft funding will be required, and will also predict how much funding is required. It is far better to have this information in advance of needing the facility, as the GP can negotiate with his or her bank from a position of comparative comfort, rather than at the time the facility is needed.

Cost–benefit analysis

In decision making, it should be appreciated that any activity has related costs and benefits. Those costs can be separated between fixed and variable costs. Fixed costs are those that do not change with the level of activity whereas variable costs do. A useful tool in decision making is contribution analysis. A contribution is defined as the difference between the income per item and the variable cost per item. The fixed costs divided by the contribution shows the number of activities required to break even.

Case example 2
Scene setting

> For example, a practice has the opportunity to reregister 2000 new patients. A registration fee of £7.10 is payable. The material costs of each registration check are £2.10. A nurse will be employed exclusively for 3 months to do the registration checks on a salary, for the 3 months, of £4500.
>
> The contribution per registration check is £5.00 (£7.10−£2.10).
>
> The number of registration checks to cover the costs of the nurse are calculated as follows
>
> $$\frac{\text{Fixed costs}}{\text{Contribution per item}} = \text{Break-even point}$$
>
> Therefore in this case, the break-even point is:
>
> $$\frac{£4500}{£5.00} = 900 \text{ patients}$$
>
> If the practice cannot register 900 patients in the 3 months, it will lose money employing the nurse. Above 900 patients, it will make money.

CONCLUSION The structure of the remuneration system at present tries to give GPs their intended average net remuneration. The present contract is more limiting than at any time in the last 15 years and there is little motivation for entrepreneurial GPs to expand their activities. This, in turn, has led to poor recruitment into training schemes, low morale in the profession, and the loss of interest and commitment in some activities that GPs have always been prepared to take on, such as 24-hour cover.

The current position cannot be maintained, and the Department of Health has perhaps two choices, to either perpetuate the current trend with ultimately the introduction of a salaried service, or to give back to the GPs the freedom and flexibility that will encourage them to develop for the benefit of both themselves and their patients. The latter option could be achieved by the local allocation of resources to GP practices by agencies familiar with their GPs, with the GPs having the discretion as to how those resources are utilized. Giving greater responsibility to the GPs would help the morale problem, which would enhance the recruitment crisis, and would ultimately lead to a more motivated profession. The former option would be a leap backwards.

SUMMARY

In order to provide an efficiency financial management system, a GP should:

♦ Have a detailed understanding of the sources of income available to the GP.

♦ Be able to use key ratios to compare the practice's financial results with average ratios.

♦ Be able to use budgets and forecasts effectively.

♦ Be sufficiently familiar with the NHS remuneration system to be able to predict and be flexible to change to protect the practice and maximize their potential.

♦ Have an understanding of how the UK taxation system operates and how it affects the practice's finances.

FURTHER
READING

♦ Chisholm, Y. (ed.) (1995) *Review Body on doctors and dentists remuneration. Medeconomics* and *GP Newspaper.* Haymarket Publishing, London.

An excellent overview of all aspects of fundholding covering both the clinical management and legal and financial side of fundholding.

♦ Pirie, A., Kelly-Madden, M. (eds) *Fundholding – A Practice Guide*. Radcliffe Medical Press, Oxford.

An independent clinical appraisal of fundholding since its inception.

♦ *Fundholding – Just what the Doctor Ordered*. Audit Commission, London.

A useful introductory guide to the GP remuneration system.

♦ *Making Sense of the New Contract*. Radcliffe Medical Press, Oxford.

An interesting and enlightening view on the future of general practice.

APPENDIX: SAMPLE SET OF PRACTICE ACCOUNTS

RAMSAY PRACTICE
PROFIT AND LOSS ACCOUNT
FOR THE YEAR ENDED 31 MARCH 1996

	Sch	1996			1995
		£	£	£	£
Fees earned (before deduction of £11 001 superannuation)	1	288 433			307 935
Reimbursements	2	333 904			288 893
Other income	3	95 767			57 009
		718 104			653 837
Less overheads					
Salaries and wages		251 056		218 354	
Staff welfare		2 267		2 974	
Locums		51 974		49 574	
Healthcall		23 277		19 598	
Drugs and instruments		14 332		8 533	
Trainee		47 992		36 311	
Courses and conferences		3 963		–	
Repairs and renewals		2 118		2 655	
Telephone		4 482		5 290	
Computer expenses		6 675		2 830	
Printing, postage and stationery		8 409		6 399	
Advertising		230		856	
Subscriptions		8 003		3 798	
General expenses		1 496		1 177	
Heat and light		3 358		2 192	
Cleaning		12 528		7 240	
Insurance		3 519		5 503	
Travel expenses		136		79	
Rent and rates		37 278		31 480	
Mortgage interest		58 414		73 671	
Training		–		688	
Book and magazines		898		296	
Room hire		–		1 220	
Rental of equipment		558		365	
Gardening and flowers		–		399	
Good health day		–		632	
Removal expenses		–		966	
Bank interest and charges		539		289	
Counsellor		175		180	
Levies		2 230		–	
Bookkeeping charges		849		–	
Legal and professional fees		7 691		–	
Accountancy		4 160		3 900	
Yoga and keepfit training		1 650		3 520	
Health centre charges		–		(4 510)	
Depreciation		8 294		6 865	
			568 551		493 324
Net profit for the year			£149 553		£160 513

RAMSAY PRACTICE
BALANCE SHEET AS AT 31 MARCH 1996

	Note	1996 £	1996 £	1995 £	1995 £
Fixed assets					
Freehold property	2		521 913		521 913
Less: mortgage			(536 011)		(535 501)
			(14 098)		(13 588)
Other tangible assets	3		26 009		30 131
			11 911		16 543
Current assets					
Fundholding Account		794		2 395	
Sundry Debtors and Prepayments		34 276		39 286	
No. 2 Bank Account		1 986		11 478	
Business Premium Account		52 603		52 260	
High Interest Business Account		–		18	
London Share Account		29 642		9 660	
Cash in Hand		168		104	
Value Added Tax		2 115		1 506	
		121 584		116 707	
Current liabilities					
Bank overdraft		27 287		2 373	
Sundry creditors and accruals		45 391		56 870	
		72 678		59 243	
NET CURRENT ASSETS			48 906		57 464
			£ 60 817		£ 74 007
REPRESENTED BY:					
Capital accounts	4				
Dr A		(4 700)		(4 530)	
Dr B		(4 699)		(4 529)	
Dr C		(4 699)		(4 529)	
			(14 098)		(13 588)
Current accounts	5				
Dr A		8 829		20 988	
Dr B		27 967		24 931	
Dr C		21 004		17 252	
Dr D		(753)		9 119	
Dr E		17 868		15 305	
			74 915		87 595
			£ 60 817		£ 74 007

RAMSAY PRACTICE
SCHEDULES OF INCOME
FOR THE YEAR ENDED 31 MARCH 1996

	Sch	1996 £	1995 £
SCHEDULE 1			
Fees earned			
Capitation fees		150 237	141 908
Basic practice allowance		27 264	29 957
Deprivation payments		208	212
Targets, Vaccinations			
Age 2: High		6 235	8 146
: Low		–	–
Age 5: High		1 783	1 676
: Low		–	217
Target, Cytology			
High		11 214	10 299
Low		–	–
Items of service	4	42 935	49 374
Child health surveillance		7 070	6 194
Registration fees		7 290	6 626
Health promotion:			
Band 3		12 506	4 760
Asthma management		1 820	875
Diabetes management		1 820	875
Minor surgery		4 965	5 556
Health promotion clinics		3 250	22 005
Transitional payments		–	2 438
Medical students		9 836	6 015
Postgraduate education allowance		–	10 156
Seniority		–	646
		£288 433	£307 935
SCHEDULE 2			
Reimbursements			
Staff		175 012	146 494
Trainee		47 992	36 311
Locums		135	7 597
Rent and rates		95 564	87 720
Computer expenses		3 637	2 095
Drugs		11 564	8 676
		£333 904	£288 893

	Sch	1996 £	1995 £

SCHEDULE 3
Other income

		1996 £	1995 £
Private fees		3 405	1 667
Training grant		6 854	3 563
Service charges income		2 998	4 285
Schedule E		18 941	12 880
Donation		–	250
Fundholding income		40 125	31 933
Good health day		–	846
Training		–	20
Sales income		22 446	–
Bank deposit interest		998	1 565
		£95 767	£57 009

SCHEDULE 4
Analysis of items of service

	Total £	1996 Per patient £	National average £	1995 Total £	Per patient £
Night Visits					
– High	96 ⎤	0.59	1.32	1 643 ⎤	0.70
– Low	5 391 ⎦			4 604 ⎦	
Temporary residents	1 815	0.20	0.36	2 352	0.26
Emergency treatment	2 825	0.31	0.04	1 722	0.19
Maternity medical services	13 243	1.44	1.45	17 277	1.93
Vaccinations	4 373	0.47	0.59	5 756	0.64
Contraceptive services	15 192	1.65	0.96	16 020	1.79
	£ 42 935	£ 4.66	£ 4.72	£ 49 374	£ 5.51

RAMSAY PRACTICE
NOTES TO THE ACCOUNTS
FOR THE YEAR ENDED 31 MARCH 1996

1. ALLOCATION OF PROFIT

		Dr A £	Dr B £	Dr C £	Dr E £	Total £
Prior allocation	£					
Cost rent	57 122					
Mortgage interest	(58 414)					
Building insurance	(1 062)					
Professional fees	(7 691)					
		(3 348)	(3 348)	(3 349)	–	(10 045)
Balance						
9.17:34.06:34.06:22.71		14 635	54 359	54 359	36 245	159 598
		£ 11 287	£ 51 011	£ 51 010	£ 36 245	£149 553

2. FREEHOLD PROPERTY

	1996 £	1995 £
Property	521 913	425 569
Property additions	–	101 488
Grants	–	(5 144)
	£521 913	£512 913

3. OTHER TANGIBLE ASSETS

	Computer equipment £	Surgery and office equipment £	Total £
Cost			
At 1 April 1995	18 006	32 423	50 429
Addition in the year	8 335	3 952	12 287
Grants	(7 051)	(1 064)	(8 115)
At 31 March 1996	19 290	35 311	54 601
Depreciation			
At 1 April 1995	8 139	12 159	20 298
Charge for the year	4 822	3 472	8 294
At 31 March 1996	12 961	15 631	28 592
Net book value			
At 31 March 1996	£ 6 329	£ 19 680	£ 26 009
At 31 March 1995	£ 9 867	£ 20 264	£ 30 131

4. CAPITAL ACCOUNTS

	Dr A £	Dr B £	Dr C £	Total £
Balance at 1 April 1995	(4 530)	(4 529)	(4 529)	(13 588)
Transfer to current account	(170)	(170)	(170)	(510)
Balance at 31 March 1996	£ (4 700)	£ (4 699)	£ (4 699)	£(14 098)

5. CURRENT ACCOUNTS

	Dr A £	Dr B £	Dr C £	Dr D £	Dr E £	Total £
Balance at 1 April 1995	20 988	24 931	17 252	9 119	15 305	87 595
Share of profit	11 287	51 011	51 010	–	36 245	149 553
	32 275	75 942	68 262	9 119	51 550	237 148
Less:						
Drawings	10 795	34 626	33 484	–	22 560	101 465
Superannuation	2 991	2 991	2 991	49	1 979	11 001
Taxation	169	6 480	10 675	704	6 826	24 854
Transfer from capital account	(170)	(170)	(170)	–	–	(510)
Repayment of capital	9 661	4 048	278	9 119	2 317	25 423
	23 446	47 975	47 258	9 872	33 682	162 233
Balance at 31 March 1996	£ 8 829	£ 27 967	£ 21 004	£ (753)	£ 17 868	£ 74 915

RAMSAY PRACTICE
SCHEDULE OF DRAWINGS
FOR THE YEAR ENDED 31 MARCH 1996

	Dr A £	Dr B £	Dr C £	Dr E £	Total £
Month					
April 1995	262	2722	2722	1836	7542
May	262	2722	2722	1836	7542
June	1140	2722	2722	1836	8420
July	–	2722	2722	1836	7280
August	1140	2722	2722	1836	8420
September	574	2722	2722	1836	7854
October	859	2722	2722	1836	8139
November	–	2722	2722	1836	7280
December	1714	2722	2722	1836	8994
January 1996	855	2722	2722	1836	8135
February	855	2722	2722	1836	8135
March	855	2722	2722	1839	8138
	8516	32664	32664	22035	95879
Endowment payments	1944	–	–	–	1944
Personal accountancy	295	295	295	–	885
Tax refund	–	1142	–	–	1142
Books	40	–	–	–	40
PGEA	–	525	525	525	1575
	£ 10795	£ 34626	£ 33484	£ 22560	£101465

RAMSAY PRACTICE
SCHEDULE OF TAXATION
FOR THE YEAR ENDED 31 MARCH 1996

	Dr A £	Dr B £	Dr C £	Dr D £	Dr E £	Total £
1993/94 refunds	–	(5395)	(3271)	704	(1133)	(9095)
1994/95 liability	169	11875	13946	–	7959	33949
	£ 169	£ 6480	£ 10675	£ 704	£ 6826	£ 24854

THE RAMSAY PRACTICE
CURRENT ACCOUNT RECONCILIATION

	Total	Dr B	Dr C	Dr A	Dr E
Balances at 31 March 1996	75668	27967	21004	8829	17868
Correct balance	75668	24327	24327	10797	16217
To repay to the practice	5291	0	3323	1968	0
To draw from the practice	5291	3640	0	0	1651

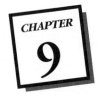

EFFECTIVE TECHNOLOGICAL MANAGEMENT

Tony Rennison

OBJECTIVES

- ◆ To understand the increasing role of information technology (IT) in the effective management of general practice.

- ◆ To show the areas in which IT can be used effectively in the management of data and to understand the associated problems.

- ◆ To provide a practical approach for the implementation of an IT strategy in practice.

- ◆ To understand the future of IT and its implications for general practice.

INTRODUCTION

Information technology in general practice is frequently misunderstood by practice members. Individuals feel that they have been left behind by the information revolution and, with all the other demands placed upon them, they cannot find the time to catch up. This is unfortunate as the *appropriate* use of IT can make a very significant contribution to increased efficiency in many aspects of the practice. This is especially true in recent years owing to the increased demands for data.

Data demands

General practice in the UK has changed greatly in the last few years and the demands for information are increasing. Targets for cytology and childhood immunizations and Health Promotion projects are prime examples of datasets which can be conveniently collected and analysed using computers. There are many more. As more practices embark on some form of commissioning, these demands are likely to increase rapidly. Unfortunately, although most practice members would accept that the above is true, often *effective management* of IT is not implemented. This leads to the situation where, for example, a particular report is needed but the output from the computer is incomplete or inaccurate, or simply cannot be obtained.

At the end of the day computers are only a tool to help primary care fulfil its role. A significant and developing part of that role is the use of information to improve both the extent and quality of patient care. GPs and their staff should be taking advantage of the potential benefits of computers, both in this respect and in order to be in control of the ever increased accountability demanded of primary care teams.

System use   The advantages of using clinical computer systems are wide ranging but can be summarized under three broad headings (Box 9.1).

Box 9.1
Advantages

- ◆ Effective administration of routine tasks, i.e. repeat prescriptions and targets.
- ◆ Maintenance of a structured, *secure* patient clinical record.
- ◆ Ability to audit and extract data, improved with *coded* data entry.

On the other hand, using a GP clinical system fully imposes some restrictions on the way practice staff work (Box 9.2).

Box 9.2
Disadvantages

- ◆ Information must be entered in the correct form and location. Data entry must be positively managed.
- ◆ Sketches and diagrams, used in the written clinical record are generally not possible at present. However, a system to be introduced soon has this facility.
- ◆ Initial time taken for data entry increases significantly.
- ◆ Significant costs will be incurred.

The use of systems will be developed in a later section but, generally, uses can be nominally split up into basic and advanced areas:

- ◆ Basic uses, i.e. registration, prescribing, targets, health promotion data, etc.
- ◆ Advanced uses, i.e. clinical data entry, referrals, pathology results, patient letters, export of data, appointments, etc.

The above differentiation is somewhat arbitrary but illustrates the point. Many practices never reach the second category of advanced use. One of the major reasons for this is inadequate time spent in selecting clinical systems.

Selecting a clinical system

A few years ago there were over a hundred suppliers of GP systems but, owing to the fact that software now has to be accredited (by the Department of Health as fulfilling certain minimum requirements), the number of suppliers actively offering software has dropped to about 25.

The selection of a GP system is by no means easy. It is often difficult to spot the strengths and weaknesses of systems in a demonstration lasting for only an hour or two. It is, however, most important that practices try as hard as possible to match their own specific requirements to a suitable system, using as many sources of information as possible. Sources include the system suppliers, health authority and other facilitators, as well as local practices – who can often be a mine of useful information.

Having selected a system, practices need to think carefully about the *hardware specification* of their new systems both in terms of the tasks and the personnel involved.

Computer hardware

Hardware is a problematical issue in general practice for a variety of reasons but the most important is the speed with which hardware becomes obsolete. For reasons of cost, hardware for clinical systems (or just stand-alone machines) are often either under-specified or marginally specified for the initial tasks envisaged. This often results in hardware being seriously inadequate after a few years. A good example of this is 'links' (Registration and IOS Claims Communication), where a large number of practices have had to upgrade relatively new systems in order to participate.

As a general principle, it is almost always a good idea to slightly overspecify hardware for a new or radically upgraded GP system, in the hope that hardware acquired in this way would remain serviceable for longer.

Other software

As well as the main clinical system, there are many types of software that can be of use in general practice. For example, standard business software such as word processors, spreadsheets, accounting packages and, more recently, Internet browsers are all examples of general purpose software which can be of great value.

As well as these, there is an increasing quantity of specialist software available including such things as distance learning packages, guides to the Red Book and specialist software for specific disease groups, i.e. diabetics.

In order to be able to use the majority of this software it is important that practices have at least one standard business personal computer (PC) either linked to their clinical system or as a stand-alone computer. Such a PC needs to be of high specification to cope with all the currently available material.

Future of Computing in general and practice computing in particular are in a
practice IT state of rapid change. Technologies are moving on at such a rate that items which were considered to be very 'high tech' even a couple of years ago are now altogether commonplace.

Suppliers are upgrading systems to use the Windows interface leading to more intuitive, easier to use programs. Advances in telecommunications are making such things as Telemedicine not only possible but commonplace. The National Health Service (NHS) network, despite a troubled birth, will be an enormous influence on many aspects of information management in the next few years.

The explosion in the accessibility of information caused by the increased use and further development of the Internet will also be likely to have a significant effect. In the future, general practitioners (GPs) will be under much stronger pressure than hitherto to make use of all the new opportunities to store, share and analyse information. Those who fail to capitalize on IT opportunities will, in all probability, find themselves at a severe disadvantage.

PRACTICE IT AND As has been mentioned, it is most important to plan data manage-
THE MANAGEMENT ment on a computer. The penalty for not taking this approach is the
OF DATA inability to extract data. Further, there will be uncertainty regarding the completeness of patient data, making the system less useful for day-to-day patient management. It is also important to consider carefully the merits of computer data entry versus manual methods and to be convinced of the benefits.

Effective management of IT in general practice is a wide-ranging subject which involves reasonably detailed analysis of why particular data are stored and what are the requirements for accessing them in the future. In essence, however, what is required is a clear understanding of what the practice is trying to achieve.

Many practices are trying to store virtually all patient data on the computer but without any systematic or clear idea of why they are doing this, other than they think that it is a 'good thing'. At some point, practices often try to extract reports on the data, for example, even a simple list of asthmatics, and find that as the whole process has not been thought through, the list cannot be produced accurately. Not unreasonably at this point people become more negative about the system and there is a tendency to say it does not work properly or that the design of the particular GP system is the problem. Clearly, the use of computers brings advantages and some potential problems.

A number of the problems are, in one way or another, concerned with clinical coding systems. As Read codes have been adopted as the standard coding system for the NHS, attention in this chapter will be confined to this coding system.

Read coding

There are two ways to store information on a computer. These are as *free text* or as an item selected from a *dictionary* or a *coding system*. For example, the term 'essential hypertension' might be used. This could be typed into a text field and stored as an unstructured data item. It is then stored as free text, meaning there is no control over the term that is entered. As a result of this many different but similar ways of entering the item could be used, i.e. 'Essential Hypertension, Essential hypertension, essential hypertension, ess. Hypertension, Ess. Hyp, etc. Data entered in this way are very difficult to search and, for this reason, coding systems have been developed. Coding systems use a particular form of expression associated with (in the case of Read codes) an alphanumeric code. The code is unambiguous and can only be stored in one form, negating some of the problems associated with free-text data entry.

The Read code system consists of various *rubrics*, which are textual descriptions of events and diagnosis, and each is assigned an alphanumeric code. It is not necessary to know the code in order to use the system, although it can make data entry quicker. Read codes, unlike a number of other coding systems, are arranged in heirarchies so that related codes are grouped together. Different *chapters* of the Read system describe different events, such as procedures, symptoms, diagnosis, etc.

One of the major advantages of this system is the ability to look at codes at different levels of detail. In general, provided items have been properly coded, it is possible to look at 'diabetes mellitus' in general or specifically at some lower level, such as 'adult onset diabetes mellitus'. The operative words in the above are *properly coded*. If several different Read headings have been used to code what is effectively one condition, then extracting useful data in bulk becomes difficult and prone to error (Case example 1).

Case example 1
Inconsistent coding

'We managed to work out how to do a search for "hypertension" but the numbers produced were far lower than expected. It turned out that Dr Y was putting on the code "blood pressure raised" rather than one of the hypertension codes and Dr Z was using "history of hypertensive disease". We hoped we could alter all the codes to one easily, but in the end we found we couldn't do that with our system. ... We had to go back and alter all the records one by one. ...'

Read codes are a major step on the road to the efficient use of computer systems in general practice but they are not without their problems. They can be slow to access, and the sheer complexity and number of codes can make them slow to use for those unfamiliar with their structure. Matters can be simplified somewhat if practices come to firm decisions on the type of data entry they wish to pursue.

Data entry   The potential use of a clinical system needs to be looked at from the viewpoint of the three main categories.

1. Effective administration of routine tasks.
2. Maintenance of a structured patient medical record.
3. Data audit and extraction.

1. Administration of routine tasks

The most widespread uses for clinical computers are for those routine everyday tasks which are well-defined and largely repetitive. This includes such items as storing and searching registration data, registration links, repeat prescribing, and entering and reporting on banding and targets and IOS claims data.

It is important to stress that, as a general principle, the aims of data entry should always be considered at every stage. For example, to search on registration status this must have been entered in all cases. Sometimes, on particular systems, details such as these are recorded as free text or not at all. Similarly, in order to be able to report which patients have had a blood pressure check, it is normally necessary to enter the blood pressure into a data field for this purpose. On some older systems, even this is not enough – it sometimes must be entered on the 'correct' screen to register in the appropriate search. With regard to drug searches, some systems allow the users to build up a dictionary of drugs and it is not uncommon for the same drug to be entered several times with slightly different spellings, etc., although again this can make searches very difficult.

In summary, the data needs to have the data entry requirements listed in Box 9.3.

Box 9.3
Data entry
requirements

♦ Consistency: record the same data in the same way.

♦ Context: make sure that entered data will register in any planned search.

♦ Completeness: ensure that data are fully entered, as partial data entry can produce very misleading results – often to the financial disadvantage of the practice.

2. Patient medical record

If the principle that a computerized medical report is desirable is accepted, then the question of what data to record and how to record them becomes relevant. To some extent this will be influenced by the nature of the medical system in use. It should also be borne in mind that the majority of systems use Read codes.

To decide if a computerized medical record is advantageous, the following questions could be addressed:

♦ In what ways are the computerized patient record superior to manual systems?
♦ Is it envisaged that the computer record will replace the paper one in the foreseeable future?

There are a number of ways in which the computerised medical record can be considered superior to its paper-based equivalent, as summarized below:

♦ Legibility
♦ Accessibility, i.e. it can be accessed from any screen in the practice.
♦ Structure, i.e. it allows the user to view the medical record in a variety of ways.
♦ Security – electronic records are both harder to access if unauthorized and easier to restore if damaged by fire, flood, etc.

There are many different levels at which data entry can be made but it is convenient to consider three different schemes (Box 9.4).

Box 9.4
Levels of data entry

♦ Full data entry – full entry of patient clinical data.

♦ Key data entry – selected entry of clinical data.

♦ No clinical data entry – only banding, target and related statutory data are entered.

Full data entry

All data that would be present in the manual notes are entered on to the computer. The main decision which must be taken is what data to Read code and what data to enter as free text.

From the aspect of *the individual patient* it does not matter how the data are entered *unless* the design of the system relies on Read coding to give structure to the clinical record (as is the case with some leading systems). Even with these systems it is debatable whether it is worth coding aspects of the medical record in great detail if coded entries can be qualified by free text.

For the individual patient record the only reason to Read code is to create structure in the clinical record. In many cases more general Read codes (higher level terms) can be used, qualified by free text. This approach will often result in quicker data entry and, therefore, tend to promote better data entry levels. This method may be modified by the desire to extract particular information at various levels of detail, i.e. for certain specified conditions such as asthma and diabetes.

Key data entry

If the entry of all data is impractical, owing to the time it would take, reluctance of principals, etc. another option is just to enter the key data. The main thing to be decided is what key data should be entered.

Major clinical events are entered to provide an effective medical summary on screen. The object is often rather more biased towards the extraction of data with the summary medical record created almost as a by-product.

This type of data entry is often easier to control than full clinical data entry as the scope of items to be entered is smaller and easier to define. This is really the only option for those practices which do not have screens in the consulting rooms and rely instead on data entered later from some form of *encounter sheet*.

Encounter sheets can be very useful provided they are easy to both complete and transcribe on to the computer, although ultimately they can act as a barrier to GPs embarking on their own data entry. A section from a typical encounter sheet is shown in Figure. 9.1.

No clinical data entry

Many practices take this path and enter no clinical data other than essential information required for banding. Sometimes this is due to the lack of functionality of the clinical system in use. Often it is due

Figure 9.1
Portion of an encounter sheet used for limited data entry

Name:	DOB:	Comp No:
Date:	GP:	Entered by:

BP / mmHg	Hypertensive dis.	Malignant Neoplasm colon
Smoking? No	Glaucoma	Malignant Neoplasm breast
Height	Reflux	Acquired Hyperthyroidism
Weight	URTI	Epilepsy
FH IHD	Cystitis	Ischaemic heart disease
FH CVA	Disorders of lipid metabolism	Inflamatory
Asthmatic PF	Rheumatoid Arthritis	Nephritis/n
Diabetic		R
Cholesterol		P
FP1001		
Lst Smear		

to a lack of knowledge on how to proceed or the feeling that vast amounts of time will be required.

With very few exceptions, most clinical systems are suitable for at least limited data entry and even the busiest or most understaffed practice should find the process worthwhile in terms of the benefits gained.

3. Data audit and extraction

The ability to extract data in bulk for patients is a powerful benefit of a properly run system. Searches and data extraction fall into two categories namely:

♦ Routine searches, such as those required for cytology and childhood immunizations, which are required at regular intervals.
♦ One-off searches (at least in the first case) to extract the identity of specific groups of patients, either as lists or sometimes with selected clinical details.

Routine searches are commonly supplied as part of the clinical system in a 'ready to go' format. This means that it should only be necessary to enter the conditions, for example, the time period for a search, in order to run it. It should not be necessary to set up the search criteria. As with all searches, however, the data have to be entered in the correct way for the search to work. In most cases, appropriate codes need to be used to enter the data.

As well as standard reports, most systems have what are normally termed *report generators* to generate reports based on complex or less common criteria. These vary widely in ease of use and effectiveness as well as the time taken to produce results.

A satisfactory report generator will allow any structured data entered into the system to be extracted in a search and some will also allow searches of free text (free text searches are to be avoided if at all possible, owing to the major problems of consistency). The latest systems split the process of searches into several distinct phases:

♦ The search – select the patients.
♦ The content – select what information should be outputted for each patient.
♦ The output format – format in which the selected data should be presented.

Despite the efforts of suppliers to make report generators both easier to use and more flexible, many practices make little use of such facilities. Initial attempts to use them are often discouraging owing to problems connected with inconsistencies in data entry or just lack of data. (Case examples 2 and 3).

Case example 2
Poor system design

> 'We had been using the ZZZZZZ system for some time and decided to pull out a list of asthmatics. We had been very careful to all use the same Read code as we had been warned about this by another practice. We were very disappointed when the results did not come out correctly. After we had talked to the helpline it turns out that Read codes entered in the "consultation" can't be searched at the same time as Read codes entered into the "Medical History" as they are in separate files. It seems a bit stupid but that's how it is. I wish we had tried out the searches at the beginning and found out about this but we just didn't know what to look for ...'

Case example 3
Completeness of data

> 'We've all been entering the health promotion (HP) data for some time and have continued as part of our HP Project. We assumed that we were getting quite a lot of data on to the machine. When I asked the partners how many patients they had entered, they all said thousands. In the event, out of 18 186 registered patients, we have HP data on 1261, which is not too good. I wish I had done the search earlier but I just assumed that it was going OK. We won't be using this data in our new HP scheme.'

Personnel management

Often problems with the implementation or use of computer systems are related to those people required to operate them. One of the basic themes running through this chapter has been the need to be clear about the reasons for using computers, but an equally important point is to make users of the system fully aware of how their contribution fits into this scheme.

An easy mistake to make is to instruct individuals on how to enter data without giving any reasons for this. A practical example of this is staff told to carefully enter information for childhood immunizations without being told how the data will be extracted. All users of a system should be aware of how searches are run so that they can fully appreciate the effect of what they do.

Another problem is those individuals who are personally opposed to using the computer at all, on principle. These can be staff or nurses or partners, but in all cases it can lead to problems. Reluctance by staff to use computers is often borne out of a feeling that in some way they are too old or unknowledgeable to use them. Positive reassurance that this is not the case coupled with encouragement for effort can usually resolve this.

The fear of GPs, if not in the above category, is often related to time. GPs often feel very pressed just carrying out their contractual obligations and are wary of becoming involved in data entry in the consultation, however clearly they can see the long-term advantages. In these cases is it often useful to try to enter data for only one or two patients a day for several months, as the time implications of this are not so severe. If this is done, familiarity with the system will lead to increases in speed of data entry so that the problem will normally resolve itself.

The specific issues related to different types of data entry at a basic and advanced level need to be considered.

BASIC USE OF SYSTEMS

Registration

Entering and using registration data is normally the first area to be explored. Generally, a download of registration data will have originally been provided by the health authority via the system supplier who will have provided the data preloaded when the system was installed.

The first task is normally to check the accuracy of these data and then maintain it as the practice population changes. Uses for the data are many but some of the most important ones are:

♦ A source of identifying information about patients.
♦ Assisting with claims – temporary residents, capitation, etc.
♦ Export of data, i.e. address, name, date of birth, etc. for patients.
♦ Searches, i.e. ages, sex, locations, etc.

Owing to the RFA (Requirements for Accreditation) rules, one registration screen tends to look quite like another and the main objective is to make sure that the various reports required by the health authority are available. Some systems have many detailed fields for information, such as mileage units and several hospital numbers. In many cases it is not particularly useful to fill in these fields.

On a recently installed system, the registration situation is often further complicated by the fact that the practice will immediately embark on registration links. Although increasing the initial difficulty of using the system, the benefits will quickly outweigh the extra complication.

Prescribing

Whereas registration data are normally handled by the practice staff, prescribing is often one of the first areas where GPs can be involved. Success in this area is normally dependent on a number of factors which include:

♦ The clinical system being user-friendly and quick in use.
♦ GPs having both computers and *printers* in their consulting rooms.

♦ GPs having the resolve (and time) to get through the first few months without giving up.

In many practices GPs become used to setting up repeat prescribing using the computer but fail ever to issue acute scripts routinely. This is unfortunate as using the computer for acute prescribing brings many benefits but, in particular, means that an accurate prescribing record is maintained for each patient. This is most useful for searches but also has benefits in terms of the individual patient record, particularly where allergies and contra-indications are set up.

Another major benefit of using the computer for all prescribing is the relative ease with which generic prescribing can be initiated. Most systems have easy methods of substituting selected brand name drugs for generics and many can totally restrict the issue of branded drugs if desired.

Prescribing is an area where there are major gains to be made by using the computer with the only possible down side being increased time taken entering scripts in the early stages.

Targets   Cytology and childhood immunization targets are probably the next items that most practices try to implement after the items described above. Nowadays, the majority of systems use Read codes to record smears/results and the various immunizations and problems are relatively rare. It is quite common, however, to find practices who have developed their own searches rather than use the routines supplied, as some find these overly complex and wasteful of paper. As has been said before, check that they work on small amounts of data before relying on them.

Most systems will now allow practices to look at targets in the future by changing the search dates. This can be very useful to try to ensure that procedures are carried out in good time to qualify for target payments. Perhaps one of the greatest problems associated with this area is to develop a foolproof recall system so that women who fail to respond to initial Health Authority generated recalls for a smear and mothers who fail to bring their children for their immunizations are 'chased'.

Overall, using computers to monitor targets is an easy and effective way to carry out this operation, and is normally vastly preferable to a manual system.

Health promotion   In the early days of health promotion banding, there were many problems with using the computer. Banding reports were not ready for the first target date even though much data had been entered and sometimes the reports did not give accurate answers. The nature of data collection for health promotion has now changed, with practices being rather more in control of the data they will collect.

ADVANCED USE OF SYSTEMS

Clinical data entry

It will be recalled that clinical data entry can take place either in the consultation or via an encounter sheet later. Sometimes a combination of the two can be used.

The main barriers to clinical data entry are shown in Box 9.5.

Box 9.5
Barriers to clinical data entry

1. Time.
2. Poor computer system.
3. Resistance to change, i.e. to change consultation methods.
4. Confidentiality, i.e. concern about electronic recording of sensitive data.
5. Maintaining two record systems.

1. Time

Time is a very important factor as initially it takes much longer to enter a consultation on the computer (and in most cases record it manually) than simply to write in the notes. The only comfort is that the process becomes a lot quicker with practice. With a good system it should be possible to enter full details of the consultation in less than about 90 seconds.

2. Poor computer system

Possessing a poor computer system can make it unprofitable to attempt to enter full clinical data and the only real answer here is to change system or restrict data entry to key items.

3. Resistance to change

GPs will often resist changes in the way consultations are carried out but in most cases GPs enter data other than prescribing after the patient has left the room. The question to be faced is: can the GP complete the data entry in the 1–1.5 minutes available?

4. Confidentiality

Security of clinical systems is, in general, quite good with it being difficult (in most cases) to extract the data without knowledge of login names and passwords. The issue is really that practices should ensure that these passwords are not widely known. Whether or not very sensitive data such as AIDS status, etc. should be recorded is a matter for individual GPs but, in general, a computer system is more secure than paper records.

5. Maintaining two record systems

The situation with regards to abandoning manual records is far from clear. To be absolutely certain of fulfilling their contracts in all situations, it would seem wise *at the time of writing* to maintain some form of written record. Some experts in this medico-legal area maintain that written records are unnecessary provided the system in use has a full *audit trail*. The audit trail provides a record of all changes made to a patient's medical record. It is certainly true that a large number of GPs have been discouraged from embarking on clinical data entry for this reason. Currently, it is a requirement of the terms of service and conditions to maintain a written record. Attention is drawn to a case in which a GP was found in breach of his terms of service because he kept only computerized clinical records. Current Department of Health negotiations are likely to legitimize electronic records in the future.

Referral entry   Entering referral data on to the computer is useful in a variety of ways, but it can take some time and many GPs are reluctant to enter the referral during surgery time. The chief benefits are:

♦ Easy production of referral letters.
♦ Easy referral analysis.
♦ Potential for data transfer to a fundholding system without rekeying.

Most modern systems are actually quite easy to use in respect of referrals *provided* dictionaries of providers, consultants, etc. have been set up. Even if referrals cannot be entered at the time of referral, it is normally worthwhile to enter the data later in order to gain the benefits. Many practices look on the entry of referral information as an advanced and difficult topic, although, in fact, analysing referrals manually is potentially more complicated.

Pathology results   There is great benefit in having pathology data for patients recorded on the system but the chief problem is the time spent entering the data. Increasingly data can be transferred from the laboratory electronically but, in cases where this is not currently possible, the potential benefits, particularly in terms of individual patient care, should be carefully assessed. The chief benefits are:

♦ Easy access to pathology data in the electronic record.
♦ Ability to look at the variation of particular results with time.
♦ Easy bulk audit of data, i.e. the control of diabetes via $HbA1_C$ values.

Against this is the fact that, in an average practice of around 8000 patients, it can take up to 0.5 person days per week to enter all the results, excluding smears.

Merging and exporting data   The ability to produce personalized letters containing data stored in the clinical system is very powerful but, in general, rather under-used. Most GP systems offer this facility but it is often fairly difficult to set up.

Unless the system is very difficult to use, it is well worth spending time and effort in learning how these features work, as generating letters to patients is much easier, quicker and much better presented than using the time-honoured method of either writing the patient details in by hand or using a photocopier. Similarly, referral letters are much easier to produce if the required clinical data is automatically or semiautomatically extracted from the computer.

Exporting data for use in PC-based software such as spreadsheets has until recently been a very technical matter in the majority of cases but it is now becoming much more common. Knowledge of how to do this can be very useful as an alternative to rekeying the data into a PC from a printed report, or even to use standard word processing for letters to patients.

Appointment systems

Appointment systems are finally beginning to be used in a significant number of practices. Early software was poorly specified and difficult to use but some of the latest systems are the reverse. There are a number of benefits to be gained from implementing an appointment system, although in some cases it requires some major changes in working practice.

The benefits of a computerized system include:

◆ Systematic control of appointments in a situation where different people are making them.
◆ Quicker access to vacant appointments.
◆ Easier access to patient records for GPs, if surgery list set up, i.e. no searching for patients during consultations.
◆ Waiting times analysis.

Although GP appointment systems have come a long way, there are still some distance from the sophistication and speed of similar systems used in other businesses, e.g. the systems used by travel agents to book passengers on to airlines.

Having considered at some length the uses of systems, we will now look at acquiring a system, either as a first system or as a change from another system.

SELECTING A GP SYSTEM

All systems have their advantages and disadvantages, but some systems are more suitable for clinical use in the consultation than others. These are the ones which have a full audit trail, making them ultimately more suitable for those practices that wish to become paperless.

The selection or upgrading of a GP system depends on many things but the following questions are probably amongst the most important to address when changes are being considered (Box 9.6).

Box 9.6
Selecting a system:
issues

- ◆ Who are the main users of the system?
- ◆ What are the most important functions of the system?
- ◆ Is the system easy to use?
- ◆ Are the costs reasonable?
- ◆ Is the support adequate?
- ◆ Is the system approved (or is approval pending) for RFA in its latest version?
- ◆ Are there enough users/sites for this system to make it commercially viable.
- ◆ Does it/will it support future requirements such as pathology links, etc.?

Acquiring information

Various sources of information on GP systems have been mentioned in the introduction but it is appropriate to supplement this by a few words on the subject of supplier demonstrations. The most common course of a demonstration is for the supplier to show the system to members of the practice and then after perhaps a few questions to leave.

To obtain the most from supplier demonstrations, consider adopting some of the following:

- ◆ Make notes on each system as you see them – this presupposes that more than one system will be shortlisted!
- ◆ Try to keep in mind those points which are most important to *your* practice.
- ◆ If possible take some degree of control of the demonstration and see the areas of the system that *you* want to see.
- ◆ Ask a lot of questions – this is a unique opportunity to have your queries answered.
- ◆ If possible try out the system. Even if you have no idea of how to use it, you may well obtain a better impression about how this system might work for you.
- ◆ Try to see the same tasks done on different systems so that you can make useful comparisons.

Hardware considerations

Computer hardware, the physical computers and other items, such as printers modems needs to be considered before purchasing or upgrading a system. Expert advice should be sought.

Computers in general practice generally fall into one of two categories. There are 'file servers' – main computers for a GP system – and 'workstations' – screens for the GP system.

Fileservers should be of high specification and generally should be overspecified for the task they are to carry out. This should ensure that they will have a useful life of at least 3 years. Buying a fileserver which is merely adequate at the time of purchase is nearly always a false economy. At the time of writing (February 1997) even a small practice should consider a Pentium 166 MHz with 32 Mb RAM and 2.0 Gb hard disk as a *minimum* specification. Workstations or stand-alone PCs can be of lower specification but the same principles apply.

GP systems are virtually always comprised of multiple screens and, in order for patient data to be available generally, some form of network is used.

There are two basic types of network:

♦ *True networks* where each screen is a computer (PC) in its own right.
♦ *Multiuser systems* where a main computer is connected directly to a number of screens. This can be either as a PC or as a 'dumb' terminal.

Which type is in use depends on the particular GP system, although there is currently a tendency away from multiuser systems towards true networks. In particular, practices should seriously consider whether the purchase of dumb terminals is cost effective in any circumstances as PCs can do all a terminal can do and also function as standard business computers for relatively little extra cost. If practices are considering a change of system, then changing from one type of 'network' to the other may mean that the building will have to be entirely rewired!

Printers, another essential hardware element often given insufficient importance in the specification of a GP system, fall into three main types:

♦ Laser – higher initial costs, but excellent print quality and cheap running costs.
♦ Inkjet – good print quality and lower initial costs than a laser printer, but higher running costs.
♦ Dot matrix – print quality poorer than above, but cheap to run and buy. Ideal for FP10 continuous paper.

Each has their place in the practice and it is important that adequate numbers of printers are present. In particular each *clinical* screen should have its own printer. Nothing deters a GP from using a computer for prescribing more than having to print prescriptions in another room and then collect them for signing.

Summary of current systems Box 9.7 lists those systems commonly available.

As well as GP clinical systems there is other software which can be run on standard business computers.

Box 9.7
Systems commonly
available

Supplier	System(s)
Advanced Medical Computers Systems Ltd*	Amysys Patient Data Management
Ambridge Business Systems Ltd	GP Manager
Brandt Computer Systems Ltd	Medico
CHIME	Paradoc, GP Care
Diya Partnership	Praxis
ECL Medical	Genprac
Egerton Medical Systems Ltd	EMIS
Exeter GP Systems	Exeter GP System
Genisyst Ltd	GRS
Hollowbrook Computer Services Ltd	Micro-Doc
ITS (Wales) Ltd	Safe Clinical System
Medical Care Systems Ltd	System 7, Meduser, MCS 2000
Microsolutions Ltd	Surgery Manager, GP Plus
Microtest Ltd	Practice Manager II
Option Software	GP7
Pennine Medical Systems	Phenix
Seetec Ltd	GP Professional
Superlink Systems Ltd	Practice Link
Network Interlinks	Smart Practice
The Computer Room	MicroMedic
Touloui Associates	Geminus
Vamp Health Ltd	Vamp Medical, Vamp Vision
M-TECH Computer Services (UK)	HMC
AAH Meditel	System 5, AMC2000, (System 6000)

OTHER SOFTWARE

Non-clinical use of computers for fundholding and general administrative tasks as well as audit and research has seen a very significant increase in the last few years. This season attempts to outline some of the major uses for computer systems other than as a clinical system. The key software areas are: Fundholding, Spreadsheets and the Windows operating system.

Fundholding

The increased take-up of fundholding by GPs has led to much increased use and availability of fundholding software. This software provides facilities to log referrals made by the practice, both in terms of clinical and financial factors, and is principally designed to manage the fundholding budget. Many of the major clinical suppliers can supply fundholding software and in many cases this can be linked to their clinical system so that referrals can be transferred from this to the fundholding system avoiding the need to enter the same information twice. As well as the clinical system suppliers, there are a number of other suppliers who specialize in this type of software, of which probably ICON is the best known.

Fundholding systems have to be accredited and this has to an extent limited the number of players in the marketplace. Those systems which are popular – Meditel, Vamp, Emis Genisys and Icon – comprise an enhanced version of the referrals system built into most major clinical systems combined with what is effectively a double entry bookkeeping system. Most have a wide range of reporting facilities. In spite of the apparent benefits of integrating the fundholding and clinical software, many practices use fundholding software from a different source and in most cases run entirely separate systems. Even in those cases where the software is from the same supplier, large numbers of practices choose to keep the two systems distinctly separate.

Fundholding software, apart from controlling the fundholding budget, contracts, etc. has the almost hidden benefit of providing the opportunity for the practice to carry out enhanced audit on the outcome of referrals. In this way the effectiveness of procedures can be measured and this can indirectly lead to improvements in patient care.

Another parallel development to full fundholding status is the development of the multifunds where a number of GPs share a fundholding budget. Software for this situation is normally based on the hub and satellite model with each GP in the multifund recording those referrels that have taken place. The central organization collates the data and controls the fund. Many multifunds are still relying on the transmission of paper between practices and the centre – a situation which is certain to change.

Spreadsheets Spreadsheets are possibly the most useful software a practice can acquire once they have a clinical system. Of course, in order to use a spreadsheet the practice must possess a PC which can operate in a stand-alone mode. The value is further enhanced if this PC can be linked to the clinical system so that data can be exported from it to the PC for use in a spreadsheet.

Spreadsheets can perform two distinct functions in a practice:

♦ Numerical calculations.
♦ Production of charts and graphs from data.

Both of these functions can be extremely useful, the first mostly in the area of practice finance and payroll, and the second as a convenient way to display the results of audit and research.

As an example of how a spreadsheet can assist the practice with finance, Figure 9.2 shows an extract from a spreadsheet for practice income.

Figure 9.2
Practice income
spreadsheet (extract)

ITEM	FEE	NO	Total FEE
BPA	£6,384.00		£0.00
Seniority 1st	£375.00	1	£375.00
Seniority 2nd	£2,500.00	1	£2,500.00
Seniority 3rd	£3,750.00	1	£3,750.00
Subtotal			£6,625.00
			£0.00
Capit 0–64	£14.60	3250	£47,450.00
Capit 65–74	£15.50	345	£5,374.50
Capit 75+	£27.50	341	£9,377.50
Subtotal			£62,175.00
			£0.00
Night visits	£45.00	23	£1,035.00
N.V. lower	£15.00	34	£510.00
Vacc 1st	£3.35	45	£150.75
Vacc Boost	£4.85	44	£213.40
Contraception	£12.75	120	£1,530.00
IUDC	£42.75	78	£3,334.50
Maternity	£159.00	21	£3,339.00
Emergency	£20.20	12	£242.40
T/R <15 days	£8.10	8	£64.80
T/R > 15 days	£12.15	77	£935.55
Subtotal IOS			£11,335.40
PGEA	£2,025.00	3	£6,075.00
Minor surgery	£100.00	2	£200.00
Reg Fee	£6.10	1	£6.10
Health PromN.	£45.00	23	£1,035.00
Child Surveill	£10.00	13	£130.00
Med Student	£10.95		£0.00

An example of a chart produced from a spreadsheet is shown in Figure 9.3.

Figure 9.3
Charting with a
spreadsheet package

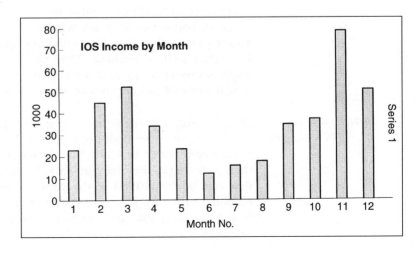

Windows operating system

PCs have traditionally used MSDOS as their operating system, and 3 or 4 years ago most software was produced to run under DOS. In the last few years, Windows and more recently Windows 95 have become popular, as these systems tend to make software more intuitive to use as well as dictating a set of common actions, making it easier to be productive with unfamiliar programs.

Windows programs are easier to use because they employ easy to follow drop down menus and prompts which can be controlled using a mouse. The consequence of all this is that software is now hugely more sophisticated than it was a few years ago and requires much more powerful computers to run it.

The net result is that, although the 'power' of computers has increased by a factor of 20 or 30 times, programs run no faster than before because of their size and vast number of features: Such is progress!

Notwithstanding the above, the future predicts massive changes in the way we all use computers.

FUTURE OF PRACTICE IT

There are a number of new developments in the area of primary health care information technology.

New generation systems

Most of the clinical systems now on the market are text based. This is partly because many systems originated at a time when most computer programs were text based and partly because of the traditional use of dumb terminals as input or output devices.

Owing to the popularity of the Windows operating environment and more recently Windows 95, virtually all the new systems are Windows based.

Of the major suppliers, Vamp have released Vision, Meditel are preparing to release System 6000 and Emis will have a Windows program soon. These new programs will have many benefits for users being easier to use and owing to extensive use of mice, less dependent on good keyboard skills.

As a consequence of being Windows-based programs, they will also require each user to be equipped with a moderately powerful PC rather than a terminal. This fact has very significant cost implications and practices will have to carefully weigh up the benefits of such systems before engaging in costly upgrades.

Future use of the NHS network

Many practices have started to use GP registration links successfully and some have continued on to items of service (IOS) links. A smaller number still have started to use electronic links with their pathology laboratory in order to receive laboratory results that can be easily filed in the patient's medical record without recourse to data input in the practice. Data entered in this way is just as amenable to searches as if data had been entered manually.

Most of these links have been effected via the RACAL wide area network (WAN) but it is planned to implement a technically more advanced WAN to be operated by Syntegra, a division of British Telecom. When this network is fully in place, it will provide the opportunity for many other types of link as well as the ones currently operating via the RACAL system. Of particular interest to GPs will be the opportunity to receive discharge summaries electronically when patients are discharged from hospital.

As well as this information, such as referral letters and other correspondence with secondary care will be sent by electronic means with all the advantages of speed, reduced workload and security.

There has been some considerable debate about the potential lack of security in the NHS network. To take a simplistic view, the system is more secure than manual records, faxes and letters which are the principal current methods employed.

Fully paperless practice

Although quite a number of practices are now paperless in the sense that they do not keep manual records of consultations, very few are truly paperless. To be truly paperless involves not only using the computer for data originating in the practice but also for items such as hospital letters coming back to the practice for patients who have been referred to secondary care.

Recently there have been developments in the integration of scanning technology which are starting to provide the solutions to make a practice truly paperless. Hospital letters and other paper data relevant to a patient are scanned using a standard scanner. The image so produced is then processed by optical character recognition (OCR) software which converts it into effectively word-processed free text. This process has not yet been perfected but is currently about 99.5% accurate. Currently some corrections are still occasionally needed after the conversion has taken place. After conversion, the file is placed, using special software, in the patient's record as a letter. Clearly this technology only works for those clinical systems which allow word-processed documents to be attached to a particular patient.

Although the development of this software still has some way to go, it should result in practices being truly paperless in the future – once all the legal questions have been resolved.

Telemedicine

Telemedicine can be defined in a number of ways but is basically the ability for individuals who are geographically in different places to participate in the same consultation. So a consultant can sit in his or her office in a hospital and, via a video or speech link, can undertake a consultation with a patient who is sitting in a GP surgery.

The technology behind this is still in its infancy and consists of a video and speech link carried between the two locations by a high-speed telephone link. The link is controlled by software running on PCs in each location with the video being captured by small video cameras mounted on top of the screens. Speech is picked up by microphones. Currently, the picture quality of the video link is poor, making it difficult to carry out effective consultations. However, the system is improving all the time as it benefits from advances in video camera technology developed for the mass market.

The technology is still rather expensive but will become cheaper as time goes on. It offers a number of benefits including more efficient use of consultant time as well as more effective involvement of the GP. From the point of view of the patient, visiting the GP is probably less stressful and more convenient than visiting an unfamiliar hospital some way away.

Speech recognition

One of the chief barriers to GPs using clinical systems is the time taken to enter data via a conventional keyboard. Recently, several products have become available which allow the user to speak into a microphone and have their speech converted into text. The main current use of such systems is in the writing of letters, which can now be dictated directly into the word processor with a fairly high degree of accuracy. In the future it is likely that the same technology will be used to enter data into a clinical system as well as control the clinical system.

Currently, the available systems recognize a particular voice with an accuracy of around 90–95%, which is not quite good enough for serious use in the consultation. Also they are very sensitive to background noise. Again the pace of development is fast and systems which are usable in primary care should be available within 2–3 years.

CONCLUSION

This chapter has tried to outline some of the fundamentals of practice computing together with a discussion of the rationale behind effective usage. The most general point that should be stressed is to plan all use of the computer and above all to test that data entry will indeed give the desired result. Although lack of success with a clinical computer system can always be attributed to the design or the support of that particular system, it is nearly always the case that much can be achieved with most of the available systems.

Practice computing is moving very rapidly, and the nature of systems and what they can do is changing in scope. Practices need to understand clearly what can be achieved with the effective use of information technology.

SUMMARY

In order to be effective in the use of information technology:

- The use of computer systems should be planned from the outset and in particular the use of Read codes.
- All staff should be aware of the reasons for using the computer and how their work fits into the entire scheme.
- PC software can be very useful particularly for word processing and spreadsheets.
- IT in general practice is changing rapidly and the new generation of GP systems are quite different from existing ones, although the specification of hardware needs to be high.
- The NHS network, although not yet fully operational, will be a major force in primary health care.

FURTHER READING

- Preece, J. (1994), *The Use of Computers in General Practice*. Churchill Livingstone, Edinburgh.

A good general text which has been the standard test for many years. A rigorous and logical approach to the subject. Biased towards general principles rather than specific systems.

- Irvine, D.S. (1991), *Making Sense of Audit*. Radcliffe Medical Press, Oxford.

Although not a book on IT as such, it is full of common sense about the rational approach to collecting data. Also covers the presentation of data using PC tools. A recommended read for anyone considering implementing new data collection in practice.

- Amery, N. (1994), Information technology. In Pine A., Kelly-Madden M. (eds) *Fundholding – A practice guide*. Chapter 10. Radcliffe Medical Press, Oxford.

A good introduction to the IT aspects of fundholding. Not system specific.

- Rennison, A.J. (1998), *A Concise Guide to General Practice Computing* (in press).

A more detailed look at the common uses of practice IT with comments on many of the major systems in use. Sections on the process of selecting hardware and software.

- *10 Minute Guides*.

Variety of volumes covering modern PC software packages from various authors. Que, Macmillan Computer Publishing. A series of basic introductory texts to common software packages such as word processors and spreadsheets. Not a lot of detail but easy to digest!

REFERENCES

Hayes, G. (1995), Primary Health Care Electronic Records – Can the technology be abused? *Proceedings of the Annual Conference PHCSG*, British Computer Society, Cambridge.

MDU (1996), Paperless records, MDU News. *Journal of the MDU* **12**:1.

NHS (1995/1996), General Medical Practice Computer Systems Requirements for Accreditation Version 3. NHS executive, HMSO.

Pringle, M., Ward, P., Chilvers, C. (1995), Assessment of the completeness and accuracy of computer medical records in four practices committed to recording data on computer. *British Journal of General Practice* **45**: 537-541.

Sullivan, F. and Mitchell, E. (1995), Has general practioner computing made a difference to patient care? *British Medical Journal* **311**: 848-852.

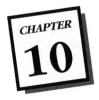

MANAGEMENT OF PEOPLE

Claire Hill

Claire Hill

OBJECTIVES

♦ To adopt an essentially 'cradle to grave' approach to managing human resources in a practice.

♦ To examine the importance of human resource planning in relation to practice planning objectives.

♦ To explore 'best practice' in staff recruitment, together with validity and reliability factors in selection and retention of staff.

♦ To assess the relevance and role of inducting, developing and appraising staff as a motivating factor in performance.

♦ To explain how to handle effectively performance and discipline problems, within the legal framework.

♦ To make clear and explain the management skills needed to facilitate the processes and procedures set out above.

INTRODUCTION During the 1990s there was much discussion and rhetoric about 'people management' or the softer techniques of management. Despite the fact that people and the way they perform absorb most of the business costs, comparatively little attention has been directed towards how to manage this valuable resource.

In general practice the emphasis has been on audit and quantitative outcomes. This chapter combines qualitative practices with quantitative outcomes because managing people effectively adds value to all businesses, not least to general practice, which is people intensive.

Managing performance problems and relationships within the practice is arguably the most difficult area of general practice. Examples of such difficulties are:

♦ Time constraints and constantly competing pressures; being forced into a reactive management situation.

♦ Small teams working closely together, making it difficult to 'step back' into a management role. Individuals involved together daily in primary care activities find it uncomfortable and unpleasant to tackle problems within the team.

♦ Contrasting and conflicting approaches between partners, leading to staff exploiting any differences.

This chapter is designed to enable a positive solution to circumvent these problems through a straightforward and proactive management approach. It deals with eliminating problems through correct management of the recruitment and selection process, i.e. getting the 'best fit' in the first place, and then explains how to manage performance effectively. Although it touches on matters of team building and employment law, these aspects are dealt with in more appropriate depth in other chapters. In summary, there is truth in the old adage that one bad apple can affect the whole barrel. Nine times out of ten, problems can be nipped in the bud if dealt with quickly, but sometimes firmer action is required where there is a continuing problem.

Getting it right leads to cost effectiveness and harmony. Getting it wrong can be a horribly expensive nightmare!

RECRUITING AND SELECTING THE BEST CANDIDATE

Why it must be right

Approximately 75% of total budget in any general practice is spent on its human resources. The importance and complexity of this huge investment is compounded by the fact that, at best, it is difficult to get rid of someone who does not 'fit in'. At worst, it is an expensive and near-impossible nightmare. Indeed, a contractual relationship should be entered into no less lightly than a not dissimilar contractual relationship – that of marriage. This is particularly true when selecting a new general practitioner (GP) partner.

Evidence abounds which suggests that more thought and preparation are devoted to purchasing a new house or car, than to recruiting a new partner, yet, unlike the partner, the house or car can be changed relatively easily. This chapter will explore tried and tested procedures and techniques to minimize the risk of a bad selection decision.

Most GPs may legitimately consider themselves to be 'a good judge of people' because they, more than most professionals, are dealing constantly with the plethora of human conditions. Perception and insight are valuable tools but are necessarily subjective, and are insufficient tools of objective measurement in the crucial investment of recruitment. Human judgement is, of course, an important part of the process but, to maximize the success of the correct decision, it must be supplemented by mechanisms for testing against predetermined and, where possible, measurable criteria. This chapter will look at what these criteria might be for different team members and how to set about assessing how people meet them.

Criteria and needs will vary from practice to practice, so the examples given are not prescriptive. Of crucial importance is the principle of the framework of assessment, which can be applied to any category of staff selection.

Since the 1980s, mounting competition and fundamental structural change in health services has necessitated the need for greater flexibility, productivity and a new ethos based on consumer satisfaction. These pressures will increase rather than diminish, and require employees to extend their skills and break down many rigidities in responsibilities and work patterns in order to shorten response times, lower costs and improve services. A *WONCA* Newsletter concluded that there was a need to 'redesign the doctor' to become 'a better communicator, a better manager, an effective educator, and able to work in partnership with patients and other service providers'. These changing needs and pressures must be reflected in recruitment decisions if general practice is to thrive and not just survive.

The trends within the profession support this view. Historically, partner turnover has been low. However, statistics show that one in seven vacancies were due to a partner leaving to join another practice and a further one in seven left to take up a new career. (Snowsie, 1992). This is indicative that additional stress factors place strains on partnerships, which, in turn, make it essential to minimize these factors at the point of selection.

This introduction has drawn on examples of recruitment of partners but the same principles apply to the primary health care team and, indeed, one bad decision in whatever functional discipline can adversely affect the whole team. The 'one bad apple' principle is a familiar one, but it must be remembered that it is often not the apple that is bad, but the selection process that places it in the barrel.

Questions to be asked and options to be explored before recruitment are shown in Box 10.1.

Box 10.1
Considerations to be explored before recruitment

> The decision to recruit is usually made as a result of someone leaving or an increased workload. At the time of a vacancy being identified, some key questions and options need to be explored.
>
> 1. The value of exit interviews.
> 2. The advantages of internal against external appointments.
> 3. To grow or not to grow.
> 4. Is job-sharing an option?

EXIT INTERVIEWS

Why has the vacancy occurred?

If the vacancy has occurred because a partner is leaving to join another practice and the implications are ignored (perhaps on the basis that he or she just did not 'fit in'), the chances are high that the same problems will be recruited into the practice in the subsequent selection process. Learning from experiences is more easily said than done. It is a salutary thought that second marriages experience a higher divorce rate simply because it is human nature to repeat mistakes. Exactly the same occurs when recruiting a new member of staff, unless present weaknesses are examined honestly and systematically, and mechanisms put in place to overcome them.

A snapshot survey in one of the larger family health services authorities (FHSAs) revealed that the policy to replace single-handed practitioners owing to retirement or ill-health, with partnerships, was failing because applicants were largely partners from existing practices who wished to work alone in order to escape the problems of working with other partners! Those partnerships that experience this problem – and these are only the tip of the iceberg – need to address the fundamental issues of why the job and that particular partnership did not measure up to the expectations of the person leaving. To think that they just did not fit in is an inadequate insurance policy against repeating a very expensive mistake which is usually unsettling for the whole team.

An 'exit interview' should be conducted with all members of staff who leave for whatever reason. Once someone has made the decision to leave, a constructive frank dialogue about their thoughts on the elements of the job, and how the role and the performance of it could be improved, provides invaluable information in deciding on what, if any, changes can usefully be made to the job, and what sort of new skills and attributes need to be recruited into it. Such an interview is usually welcomed by the outgoing person who likes having their views sought and is, after all, the person best placed to offer an opinion on that particular role. It needs to be conducted in an informal, non-judgemental and fact-finding way.

Exit interviews provide a wealth of useful factual information which is the first building block in the recruitment process. Ideally, they should also be the basis of honest scrutiny about such things as the adequacy of communication and mutual support in an increasingly pressurized profession.

AN INTERNAL OR EXTERNAL APPOINTMENT?

The value of an internal appointment, e.g. to the post of practice manager, is clear in terms of:

♦ Advertising costs.
♦ Management time in the recruitment process.
♦ Job training.

♦ The time taken to become familiarized with the organization.
♦ Improved staff motivation.
♦ Team development.

However, at the time the vacancy occurs, thoughts need to be concentrated not on a possible known person to fill it, but on the expanding role or demands of the job, and the skills and abilities which would maximize its overall contribution to the work of the practice. If the starting point is to think of the person who could fill it, this limits the scope and potential of the role within the team, and can limit creativity and innovations which will benefit the organization. A cardinal rule should be: make sure the person fits the job, not the job the person!

A job awarded on the basis of time served, reliability and a known pleasant personality could severely limit the development and potential of the practice if the necessary skills do not exist at the higher level requirement. If these are tested in open competition, the satisfaction of the job holder will be far greater and the process of objective measurement will gain the respect of the other team members, including any unsuccessful internal candidate, provided they are given constructive feedback and are not allowed to view it as a negative experience.

TO GROW OR NOT TO GROW?

Organizations have learned that to expand and grow in terms of numbers does not always bring proportional benefits. The larger the business, the more difficult it is to communicate with the component parts because communication is time, which is an expensive and precious resource. Communication is usually the first casualty when under pressure, and yet it is the lifeblood of all successful organizations.

Larger practices could usefully take stock if a partner is leaving. Could this be an opportunity to reduce list size incrementally and, perhaps, increase the cohesion of the practice? Do the benefits of enlarging outweigh the present situation? Will more partners mean less control and less team spirit?

Costs (not just financial) and practice income need to be carefully weighed in order to achieve the correct balance. If the 1980s taught us any lesson, it is that expansion as a general principle is ill thought out.

A key to a successful business is how to use human resources most effectively. This increasingly means the breaking down of traditional functional barriers and job enlargement. This applies equally to the medical and nursing professions, both of which traditionally can become entrenched in lines of demarcation.

In the case of a GP vacancy, as an alternative to traditional recruitment, it might be considered appropriate to appoint an additional practice nurse whose main activities would be to meet practice targets in immunization and cervical cytology, thereby freeing up the time of the GPs in the practice who habitually had to dedicate their time to these routine areas.

The issues of professional demarcation will continue to be a hot potato, but are worthy of further debate and educational training in increasingly pressurized times.

A person who will not or cannot delegate is a bad manager, and is destined to suffer the same fate as the dinosaurs.

IS JOB-SHARING AN OPTION? The difference between job-sharing and part-time work is commonly confused, thus the benefits of dividing a whole post between two people are often overlooked. It is a frequently held view that a 'full-time' job, whether it be that of a nurse, a doctor or a practice manager, cannot be divided up between two people, or that to do so would prove messy and complicated.

This view defies the evidence and the facts which are as follows:

1. A job shared provides the organization with two people for much the same cost as one.
2. Two people, each only working half the normal number of hours, usually bring more productivity and creativity, with a greater total input of energy into the job than one person could mentally or physically contribute.
3. It provides the opportunity to recruit into the practice complementary skills and strengths, which one person, however able, might find difficult to bring.
4. It can reduce the need for discontinuity of service and outside locum cover at times of leave or sickness, if the job share partner covers negotiated absence periods.

Whilst there are proven benefits in terms of productivity and energy levels, the decision to take on two people rather than one, needs to be considered very carefully. The recruitment processes described shortly, involving breaking a job down into component parts and analysing the skills needed to perform it, are particularly vital for a job-share situation in order to recruit complementary skills and experience, and maximize the contribution to the work of the practice. It is, of course, crucial, that the two job-holders have above-average communication skills. The key to a successful job-share is firstly, complementary interests/skills/abilities and, secondly, an ability and willingness to interact and communicate closely with the job-share partner in order that the 'seams' do not show, or are minimized.

The only jobs which cannot be shared are generally those involving a training scheme where splitting a job would clearly not be viable.

To avoid any misunderstandings, the contracts of employment for job-sharers need to specify how they divide the working week.

It may be appropriate to include a work 'overlap' to enable a handover or to cope with peak work periods.

When job-sharers do extra hours to cover their partner's absence, this has traditionally been reimbursed as flat-time rates, rather than overtime rates, until such time that the number of hours worked exceed the normal full-time hours. However, this could be disputed as discriminatory under national and European laws, and normal overtime rates, where applicable, should be considered.

Benefits, such as pay and holiday entitlement, should be divided in proportion between the hours worked. Job-sharers are only entitled to statutory sick pay if they are sick on a 'qualifying day', i.e. a normal working day and the first three qualifying days of incapacity for work are disregarded. However, employers and employees are at liberty to agree what days will be 'qualifying days'.

It is useful to consider a job-share option when a valued female member of the practice team wishes to leave or reduce her hours in order to cope with family responsibilities. The costs to the practice of losing trained and tested members of staff can far outweigh the perceived disadvantages of a job-share partnership and all options should be considered.

JOB ANALYSIS AND DESIGN

This is the first step in the recruitment process and simply involves being absolutely clear about the precise elements of a job. If you are not absolutely clear on this, you will not subsequently be able to assess performance adequately and, indeed, it could lead to the new recruit's perception of the role being different from your own expectations. The potential for future difficulties with a member of staff are emerging even at this stage! However, the scope for a mismatch can be minimized through the process of identifying the various tasks, duties and responsibilities, and then identifying the skills, abilities and experience needed to match the duties defined.

This process of analysis enables one to think through the job, reflect any changes, and make the role more effective for the practice and more satisfying for the future post holder. Offering staff satisfying, well-designed jobs will minimize turnover, increase motivation and performance and make the organization more competitive (Box 10.2, p. 232).

A good starting point for job analysis is the exit interview process described on page 228. As part of this, it can be very useful to ask the outgoing staff member to list the job duties and then attach a rating to each, denoting time against importance. This helps place in perspective the proper priorities of the job, but also identifies how the time available is actually spent. It can throw up some surprising (and even depressing) results. It is also an excellent basis to reevaluate priorities against time management and take stock of practices that have developed in an unplanned or uncontrolled way. An example of such a job-analysis tool is shown in Figure 10.1,

Box 10.2
Elements of a well-designed job

The Advisory, Conciliation and Arbitration Service (ACAS), in its Advisory Booklet: *Recruitment Policies for the 1990s*, states that the factors that make up a well-designed job vary but, in general, satisfying jobs should contain at least some of the following elements:

♦ A variety of pace and method of working, work locations and skill level.

♦ Formation of a coherent whole and provision of a visible contribution to the organization's product or service.

♦ Allowance to employees of some discretion and control in the timing, sequence and pace of work.

♦ Provision of clear and challenging job goals, and inclusion of some responsibility for outcomes.

♦ The offer of opportunities for development and advancement.

♦ The enabling of employees to contribute to decisions affecting their jobs and objectives.

and, indeed, it can be a salutary and useful experiment for all members of the practice to carry out, even if they are not leaving.

THE JOB DESCRIPTION AND PERSON SPECIFICATION

Once this process has taken place and the job has been reassessed or redesigned to pick up any deficiencies, and reflect organizational changes, a job description should be drawn up describing the main responsibilities and tasks.

A simple proforma can be used for this, based on the ACAS codes of practice recommended by employment law. This will be a straightforward task because the content of the job description has already been decided as a result of the analysis exercise. However, the job description is very important because:

1. It is the document which is given to applicants and, therefore, creates an impression of an organization.
2. It gives vital information to those who will be interviewed and to the person who is ultimately appointed.
3. It can act as an essential neutral arbiter in the case of a subsequent dispute over job content.
4. If someone were either to be dismissed or leave and then claim unfair dismissal, an industrial tribunal would expect the management to produce a job description and it can be the key part in the defence of a case.

Figure 10.1
A job analysis tool

Job title
Main role of job
Main duties
List the duties in the space provided and then, using the scale of importance given, rate each one and note the time taken to carry it out.
Importance

	1	2	3	4	5
	Very little	Low	Average	High	Vital

Percentage of total time taken

	Under 10%	10%–30%	30%–60%	60%–90%	Over 90%

Duties	Importance	Time taken

5. It is an interviewer's vital tool, in that it decides the person specification, which defines the characteristics the post holder must have to do the job, i.e. a description of the skills, qualities and experience required.

The purpose of the job description is to provide a clear picture of the job for both the practice and applicants, whilst the person specification is a tool for ensuring the best match between the applicant and the standards expected.

Without careful analysis a job description could be, at worst, inadequate or misleading and, at best, mean different things to different people. As a consequence, the skills and qualities needed could be wrongly identified in the person specification and an inappropriate person appointed.

The process of drawing up the job description and person specification can be as valuable as the purpose of the exercise itself because it requires as many participants as appropriately possible to contribute their views about the job and qualities needed. This is a useful communication exercise in that it involves, ideally, a cross-disciplinary approach, the seeking of views and discussion and, eventually, a broad level of consensus. The immediate and long-term advantages of this are two-fold:

1. People become more motivated when they are involved in the decision-making processes. They will be more committed to the ultimate success of the post and post-holder if they have had an input into the recruitment to it. This can be a valuable teambuilding exercise in itself.
2. Particularly, although not exclusively in the case of a GP vacancy, the process described will usually identify any areas which provide scope for disagreement among the partners. More importantly, it provides the mechanism to resolve them. Agreeing to adhere to a recognized procedure which is as objectively designed as possible, can be a sound basis for depersonalizing issues or small irritations that have existed often covertly, for a long time. It provides the means to overcome differences in perception, by focusing on the issues, not on personalities.

For example, the scenario of a GP joining a practice, only to leave within a relatively short space of time is unfortunately not an unfamiliar one. Almost invariably in this situation, the objective analysis and skills identification described, will not have been carried out. The interview is often rather perfunctory and one-sided, the reason being that the partners have not communicated and achieved a good consensus amongst themselves, let alone sought the views of other interested parties, such as the practice nurse or midwife. The lack of communication can be to avoid unearthing problems or differences which are known to exist. Sometimes the interviewee picks up that all might not be ideal in this practice, but accepts the job because other factors are right, such as location etc. However, plastering over any cracks at this stage is short-term expediency with, perhaps, long-term costs if the new recruit finds himself or herself in a role which has not been adequately defined and agreed, and is unable to influence existing relationships and patterns of communication to mutual satisfaction.

The standard models of a job description and person specification, as recommended by ACAS, are set out in Figures 10.2 and 10.3 and are followed by some generic examples of how these might be used to look for three roles within a practice team (Figures 10.4–10.8). The samples are intended to be neither prescriptive nor exhaustive, but simply an illustrative and useful guide.

Figure 10.2
Job description
proforma

1. Job title. 2. Main purpose of job (to be described in a single succinct statement). 3. Main duties (list tasks and responsibilities). Source: ACAS (1990)

To Figure 10.2 might usefully be added:

4. Responsible to (e.g. practice manager in the case of a receptionist).
5. Accountable to the practice partners.

These addenda indicate that direct reporting lines and overall accountabilities are not necessarily one and the same thing.

Figure 10.3
Person specification
proforma

	Essential	Desirable	How attributes are classified
Impact on other people			Appearance, speech and manner
Qualifications and experience			Education, training, experience, skills
Innate abilities			Initiative, apititude for learning
Motivation			Consistency, determination and success in achieving goals
Adjustment			Ability to stand up to stress and work pressures; ability to get on with different people

Source: ACAS (1990), based on the Munro–Fraser five-fold classification system.
N.B. The Qualifications and experience box might usefully be broken down to two for professional staff: qualifications and training and, secondly, experience and skills.

In drawing up the person specification, it is important to bear in mind that one is identifying knowledge and aptitudes that can be tested, wherever possible, through the interview process or through simple tests. For example, a common weakness is to state: 'above average intelligence'. This begs the question, what is 'average' intelligence, and how is it tested? It is more useful to define the competencies required in the context of the job. This information will form the basis of an accurate, informative advertisement and a sound selection procedure. It will also help to eliminate different and, perhaps, conflicting views of the tasks which the post holder will perform. The work required at this stage is simply a natural progression from the job analysis and

---

JOB DESCRIPTION

Job title: Practice manager

Location:

Responsible to: The Partners

Responsible for: Practice staff

Main purpose of the post:
To manage and administer the work of the practice office in accordance with the highest professional standards and in accordance with the policy and instructions of the partners, in the best interest of the partnership and the patients of the practice.

Major duties and responsibilities
1. Management of staff
2. Administration of practice finances
3. Practice organization
4. Health and safety
5. Management of premises
6. Any other reasonable duties within the capability of a practice manager.

Specific tasks:
1. Management of staff
◆ To ensure all staff have contracts, job descriptions, understand the procedure for disciplinary and grievance and performance appraisal.
◆ Provide the full range of personnel management services: selection supervision, training, welfare, health and safety, disciplinary and grievance procedures and delegation of work loads for all members of practice staff.
◆ To organize the duty rota of practice staff (including holidays and other leave) to provide an efficient service to the partners and patients.
◆ Liaise closely with all other members of the primary health care team.

2. Administration of practice finances
◆ Control, calculate and prepare practice staff (Sage payroll) and trainee salary including PAYE, NIC, SSP, SMP, pension schemes. Trainee vehicle allowance and procedures for reimbursement.
◆ Maintain and calculate practice finances monthly.
◆ Control and record petty cash.
◆ Complete and forward end of year tax returns on practice staff.
◆ Ensure submission of claims and check receipt of payments to and from health authority.
◆ Liaise with accountant, bank and health authority.

3. Practice organization
◆ To coordinate the day-to-day work of the staff employed by the practice to provide an efficient service to the partners and patients.
◆ Arrange for the purchase of refreshments, stationery, medical/cleaning supplies and sundry items either directly, or by delegation to another member of practice staff.
◆ Liaise with practice staff on changes within the practice, making sure these are implemented.
◆ To attend and minute practice meetings.

4. Health and safety
◆ Produce health and safety policies and procedures.
◆ Train staff on health and safety policies and procedures.
◆ Ensure premises and staff insurance is maintained.
◆ Ensure all accidents or dangerous incidents are investigated, recorded where necessary and any follow-up undertaken.

5. Management of premises
◆ Ensure adequate cleaning, safety, fire prevention and general maintenance and security of the premises.
◆ Train staff and delegate responsibility for general security of the premises.

6. To perform any other task*
As required, appropriate to the role of a practice manager.

*N.B. A 'catch-all' phrase can be useful but, in the event of any dispute, the law always applies the test of reasonableness, i.e. what additional duties is it *reasonable* to ask the post-holder to undertake, in the light of their skills and training.

Figure 10.4
Sample job description for practice manager

Figure 10.5
Sample person
specification – practice
manager

	Essential	Desirable
Impact on others	Open, approachable disposition A good communicator A good listener Tidy appearance	
Qualifications and experience	Experience of: financial management, staff supervision, basic personnel procedures, liaison with outside bodies, working to tight deadlines and priority-setting	A management qualification, e.g. in finance or personnel. Experience in negotiation. Knowledge of health and safety requirements. Computer-literate
Innate abilities	Clear, logical approach to problem solving, a high level of initiative, practical, good organization skills Flexibility	A good sense of humour
Motivation	Enthusiasm and determination in achieving goals. Knowledge or experience in how to motivate others and create a team spirit	
Adjustment	A robust and versatile disposition which can cope with fluctuating pressures and deal with stress in self or others. Knowledge or experience in how to deal with situations involving conflict. Good health and attendance record	

description stages already described, but accuracy is essential if the defined needs of the practice are to translate into a successful appointment.

THE ADVERTISEMENT   It is easy to write an imprecise or poor advertisement. The first symptoms of such a mistake are usually an avalanche of applications, over 50% of which are totally unsuitable, but all of which must be trawled through, incurring time and effort.

It is important neither to understate nor overstate the skills and qualifications sought. Understatement will raise the hopes of unsuitable candidates and waste the selectors' valuable time in

Figure 10.6
Sample job description
– medical receptionist

Job title: Medical receptionist
Location:
Responsible to: Senior receptionist
Responsible for:
Main purpose of the post: To provide a point of contact for patients and act as a focal point of communication between patients, doctors and other medical staff.
To ensure that:
1. Enquiries from patients, doctors and other medical staff are efficiently and courteously handled.
2. The filing, record keeping, and distribution of documents is undertaken efficiently and promptly.
3. The surgery premises are kept tidy.
4. The doctors' clinical procedures are handled efficiently.
Main duties and responsibilities
1. Opening and closing the premises.
2. Restoring telephone services.
3. Distributing patients' records to the doctors for their surgeries and ensuring that the records of any patients without appointments are available to the doctor when the patient is seen.
4. Receiving and routing patients on arrival.
5. Answering general enquiries, explaining surgery procedures. Making new and follow-up appointments, and receiving requests for repeat prescriptions.
6. Filing and extracting records and any documents relating to these including:
(i) Filing records of new patients received from the health authority.
(ii) Extracting records or withdrawals from list to send to health authority.
7. Receiving and transferring requests for home visits.
8. Receiving messages for nurses.
9. Ensuring that an adequate supply of stationery is available in the consulting rooms and the examining rooms.
10. Ensuring that an adequate supply of medical equipment is available in the consulting rooms and the examining rooms.
11. Ensuring that consulting rooms and examining rooms are kept tidy and cleared after surgeries.
12. Ensuring that records and any documents relating to clinical procedures are extracted and completed.
13. To chaperone patients if required by the doctor in surgery and during clinical procedures.
14. Making tea or coffee for the doctors.
15. Opening and distributing the mail.
16. To perform any other task as required, appropriate to the role of a medical receptionist.

Figure 10.7
Person specification –
medical receptionist

	Essential	Desirable
Impact on others	Open, friendly disposition. Good verbal communication and listening skills. Tidy appearance	
Qualifications and experience	Experience of routine administrative tasks, i.e. record-keeping, filing, maintaining systems. Good telephone answering skills	Any course or qualification involving dealing with the public or customer care. Previous experience of primary care. Computer literate
Innate abilities	Initiative and common-sense. A sense of humour.	
Motivation	Enthusiasm for the job. A positive wish to work as part of a team. An interest in the work of a PHCT	
Adjustment	A flexible disposition which will withstand pressurized situations. An ability to deal with competing demands and remain calm and courteous when under pressure. Good health and attendance record, punctuality	Knowledge of local community, e.g. any special factors such as ethnic groups. Lives locally.

Box 10.3
Rules for writing a
good advertisement

The simple rules for writing a good advertisement are as follows:

1. Job title.
2. Location.
3. Rewards offered (salary and any other benefits).
4. Brief description of organization.
5. Brief description of the job.
6. Minimum essential skills and abilities required.
7. Method of application and closing date.

Figure 10.8

Sample job description – practice nurse (for grade F post)

Hours of work . . . .

Post holder is accountable to the UKCC and . . . as the employer

Job summary

The post holder is required to provide skilled nursing care to the practice population working within practice protocols. He/she will be working independently in identifying, implementing and evaluating the nursing care given to individuals. He/she will have responsibility for implementing Bank III health promotion requirements, and will be involved in development of future services to the practice population.

Job description

The post holder will initiate and manage a programme of cardiovascular disease prevention for individual patients liaising with other members of the primary health care team where appropriate. The programme will be run within agreed protocols which he/she will assist in developing.

The post holder will initiate and manage a programme of nursing care for clients with the following chronic conditions: e.g.

1. Diabetes
2. Asthma

Management of the conditions will be within agreed practice guidelines and the post holder will liaise with other members of the primary health care team where appropriate, ensuring that the care of the client is facilitated through communication with other members of the primary health care team. He/she will have responsibility for evaluating programmes of care for individuals and will contribute to the audit and review of the guidelines.

The post holder will seek to develop new initiatives for the prevention of ill health, with regard to the targets set out in *The Health of the Nation*.

The post holder will provide the following skilled practical procedures independently to the practice population:

Suture removal, ear syringing, management of minor injuries, cervical cytology and travel immunizations, making sure that they maintain high professional standards and work within the UKCC Code of Professional Standards and work within the UKCC Code of Professional Conduct and UKCC Scope of Professional Practice.

He/she will implement, monitor and maintain an infection control policy which meets agreed standards and will work within health and safety legislation.

He/she will help to develop and review practice guidelines and protocol.

He/she will ensure that nursing intervention is regularly audited within the practice.

He/she will be able to continue their professional development in line with UKCC requirements and the needs of the practice population.

The post holder is part of the primary health care team and will attend meetings etc., relevant to maintaining strong links with other members of the primary health care team.

This job description may be reviewed and changed at the discretion of the employer and in consultation with and the agreement of the post holder.

Source: Essex FHSA

Figure 10.9
Person specification for grade F practice nurse

	Essential	Desirable
Skills and knowledge	RGN, asthma and diabetes courses. Awareness of legal and accountability issues. Regular continuing education	Family planning/cervical cytology courses. Nursing audit/ knowledge. Computer literacy
Work experience	At least 2 years practice or community nursing experience within last 5 years. Evidence of using own initiative	Previous work in general practice or as part of a team within NHS. Teaching experience. Infection control
Personal qualities	Enthusiastic. Eager to learn. Pleasant. Able to work independently. Aware of professional limitations. Uses common sense	

Source: Essex FHSA.

eliminating such applications. Overstatement will discourage perhaps the ideal candidate from applying.

'Self-selection' will take place, thus saving the interviewer's time, if the key essential elements from the person specification are included in the advertisement.

Employment law and good practice require that no terminology is used which could imply discrimination, which could be on grounds of sex, race, marital status and disablement.

Once again, the key is to concentrate on the essentials of the job in order to avoid making any value judgements about the person required. For example, people with very regular domestic responsibilities will not apply for a job which clearly states that flexibility in working hours is required. If the advertisement and job description are clear on the matter of hours and flexibility, there is no need for the selectors to even ponder about family responsibilities or childcare arrangements.

Although any implications about preferred gender or race in an advert is unlawful, there are exceptions to this rule under the Sex Discrimination Acts 1975 and 1986, and the Race Relations Act 1976. The nature of the work in general practice means that this exception could occasionally apply, specifically on grounds of 'genuine occupational qualification' (GOQ) for reasons of 'decency'. These situations only arise when a person's gender is essential to the work role. For example, the medical receptionist job description states 'To chaperone patients if required by the doctor in surgery and during clinical procedures'. Where this is a genuine and essential requirement, it would be permissible to state

Figure 10.10
Sample advertisement
for GP partner

Location: Replacement partner for group practice established for more than 40 years in this successful new town. Four full-time/two job-share partners with 10 900 patients living in compact, urban practice area with good communications and support facilities, purpose-built health centre providing accommodation for core primary health care team and for other staff such as dietician, chiropodist, relate counsellor, physiotherapist and community mental health team.

Full complement of ancilliary staff, practice computer (AMSyS). Good local hospital facilities with open access for pathology, radiology and physiotherapy, local GP maternity unit, comprehensive postgraduate programme.

Hardworking, democratic, fundholding partnership with higher than average income. GP cooperative covering out of hours service.

Closing date for applications ...

Vacancy from ... but willing to wait for suitable applicant. Details about the practice and the town will be sent to those on our initial shortlist.

Reply with personal details to Dr G. Smtih and partners.

Address ...

that a female is required, and this should be qualified by stating that it is a GOQ under the terms of the Acts. However, this would not be a valid defence if there are already an adequate number of females in the practice who can perform this function.

Similarly, a practice which has a significant ethnic minority population may legitimately specify a female GP is required if cultural or religious convention requires that a male may not examine females from that group.

If gender or race is considered to be a legitimate consideration in the selection process, the Equal Opportunities Commission or the Commission for Racial Equality can be contacted for free and independent advice, to avoid any legal pitfalls.

The sample advertisement above (Fig. 10.10) for a GP replacement meets the criteria described and refers to an information pack to be sent to shortlisted applicants. It should not be forgotten that selection is a two-way process and that advertisements serve an important public relations function. In times of a plentiful supply of applicants, such good practice has often been overlooked. However, at a time when, for example, the GP recruitment market is not as ebullient as it was some years ago, it is essential to 'sell' the benefits of the practice and see selection as a genuine two-way process. This should be standard good practice even in areas which anticipate no recruitment shortages.

THE INFORMATION PACK – CONTENTS AND ADVANTAGES

It is recommended that an information pack be compiled for GP partners and for practice managers. This not only gives an excellent impression to candidates (bearing in mind that a number of practices may be competing for the best applicant), but it also gives candidates the opportunity to 'self-select'. This self-elimination process is valuable because partners will not have to interview candidates who only find out on the day that either they are unsuitable for the practice, or the practice is unsuitable for them. The experience half-way through an interview of 'What am I/is this person doing here?' is, indeed, a dispiriting waste of time and energy for both parties. The following are examples of where additional information can be useful.

(a) Where the practice is situated in new towns, such as Harlow or Runcorn New Town, or in an inner-city area, where the benefits of living near the practice area may not appear immediately attractive. People's perceptions are often erroneous, based on scant information and, in this situation, it is advantageous to send applicants some examples of property details, including prices, in the surrounding areas. The thought of spacious, elegant Victorian villas or close rural areas will often lend new insights to previous misconceptions.

(b) Where the practice has a preferred persuasion in the form of religion or politics, this needs to be made explicit, preferably in the advertisement and certainly in the information pack, in order for unsuitable applicants to self-eliminate.

(c) Where the practice has a policy of shared care in ante- and postnatal work, involving GP unit or home deliveries, this needs to be clearly understood by all candidates. Seemingly sound applicants can often withdraw at the offer stage of the selection procedure, simply because such a policy was not made sufficiently clear until the actual interview, and their clinical experiences does not equip them sufficiently to contribute to such a policy.

The information pack should contain:

1. Information about the practice, e.g. total list size, nature of population served, details of support team and facilities, whether a training practice, philosophies and policies.
2. Information about the town/locality/surroundings, including examples of properties and schools.
3. Information about aptitudes, expectations, skills and values which are relevant to the job, both short and long term. This is not the onerous task it might seem, because the identification of essential attributes has already been done in the planning stage, in the form of the person specification. Indeed, its inclusion in the pack will satisfy this requirement and will be the best basis for applicant self-selection.
4. Information about the selection process, i.e. who is involved, selection method(s), dates and time anticipated to complete the process.

5. An invitation to send a self-assessment supporting letter based on what the candidate has learned about the practice philosophies or policies. (This could take the form of a specific question which the candidate is asked to address in no more than two sides of A4 paper.)

Potential candidates will now have had an opportunity to:

♦ Learn about the expectations of the practice.
♦ Assess their abilities and aspirations against these expectations.
♦ Decide, as a result of the above, whether to pursue the application and submit a supporting document together with their application or curriculum vitae (CV).

A proportion of those who originally responded to the advertisement will self-select out at this stage, either because they are not compatible with details provided or because of the effort involved. However, those candidates wishing to pursue their application, will do so in the full knowledge that there is a serious interest on both sides, and that the practice had put time, thought and effort into recruiting a partner who will be able to fulfil a satisfactory and satisfying role.

The above reflects the two-way nature of the process, whereby neither party wastes the time nor expectations of the other, leading to a mutually acceptable conclusion.

APPLICATION FORMS, CVs OR LETTERS OF APPLICATION

There is no single best way of inviting applications, but there are definite advantages in determining the method of application depending on the job advertised.

For the selectors, referencing particular sections is far easier than searching through sheets of individually organized letters or CVs. Application forms make it relatively easy to locate relevant pieces of information linked to job criteria. Apart from containing standard personal information, application forms can easily be produced to reflect the categories of the person specification such as (e.g. in the case of a practice manager):

♦ Experience in managing finance.
♦ Experience in managing people.

(and half a page should be allowed under each heading).

In this way, the essential elements of the person specification that can be assessed at the application stage can be transferred as headings of the application form. This eliminates superfluous detail and streamlines the selection process. Of course, only certain essential criteria can be gleaned from the application form. This will need to be further explored at interview, as will relevant interpersonal skills which clearly cannot be assessed from a written application.

Box 10.4
Benefits of using
application forms

- ◆ They make it easier to compare like with like.
- ◆ The employer determines what information is included.
- ◆ The information obtained can be used as the basis for interview.
- ◆ It can be easier for applicants to complete an application form than to write a letter.

Source: ACAS (1990)

Advantages of the CV and written letter of application are that it might reveal more of the applicant's personality. However, this is a less job-focused approach and personality can better be brought out at interview.

Whatever format is decided upon, remember that the method of application chosen should be the one which allows the selectors to match skills and experience to the person specification as accurately as possible and to cut down on processing unnecessary paper work.

SHORTLISTING After the procedures described, the number of unsuitable applications received should be reduced through the self-selection/ elimination process. The applications received now need to be reviewed systematically, and this is most easily done using a short-listing form which indicates the essential attributes highlighted in the person specification. Some essential elements can be identified from the application form, but many will need to be tested at later stages. In the case of a practice manager, the shortlisting form could look as shown in Figure 10.11.

This can considerably streamline the process of sifting through a large number of applications and produce a viable shortlist of no more than six candidates based on the essential requirements of the job, which can be identified at this stage.

Figure 10.11
Sample practice
manager shortlisting
form

Criteria	Candidates									
	1	2	3	4	5	6	7	8	9	10
Experience of supervising staff										
Financial/budgetary experience										
Supervising/management qualifications										
Etc.										

REFERENCES References are a woefully neglected area of the selection procedure, either because they are not sought at all or because the
information requested is inadequate. However, referees will normally respond positively to specific requests for information.

Information is usually sought about the applicant's honesty,
reliability and time-keeping, together with the views of the present
employer about the person's suitability for the post under consideration, leaving the onus on the present employer to choose
what may be relevant and, more importantly, what to leave out.

To overcome this, the person specification, or perhaps six key
points from it, should be sent to the present or past employer,
asking them to address their comments specifically to these main
aspects of the job. This will supply relevant and focused, instead of
generalized, information. The present employer should also be
asked about the number of days sick absence the applicant has
taken in the previous 12 months and whether they would re-
employ the person.

**SELECTION
METHODS AND
THEIR VALIDITY** All methods of assessment should be, as far as possible, reliable and
valid. Reliability means getting the test right and validity means
getting the right test. Figure 10.12 shows the validity of various
methods. The use of personality tests and assessment centres are
rising but the picture remains much the same, demonstrating that

Figure 10.12
Selection methods and
job performance

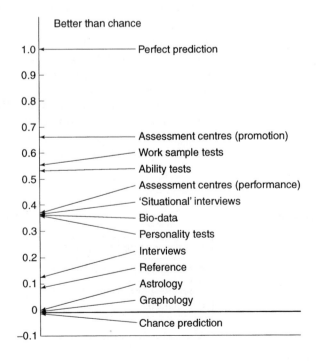

interviews are the most common *sole* method, despite a very low rating when used as the only indicator of job performance. The highest ratings are attributed to cognitive tests, involving the candidate demonstrating a practical understanding of issues relevant to the job, and assessment centres where candidates undergo several job-related assessments, including an interview. The most valid indicators of future performance are, therefore, forms of assessment which are based on the job competencies which have already been identified in the person specification.

OCCUPATIONALLY RELEVANT ASSESSMENT

Tests used as a means for measuring competencies in the job need to be thought through and used carefully in order to be valid indicators. No single test, including an interview, should be viewed as a single satisfactory indicator because the whole range of the person specification cannot be assessed from one test alone.

Attainment tests

These are designed to measure specific knowledge or skills in a particular area. Examples of this could be setting a timed keyboard exercise for a typist or computer operator, or a sample budgeting exercise for a job which involves handling the budget or numerical acumen.

Aptitude and trainability tests

These are designed to measure specific capabilities and indicate what a person is likely to attain in the future, rather than measure what has already been learned. These could include placing someone in a simulated counselling situation to assess their listening and facilitation abilities, or give them a problem-solving exercise which will provide an indication of the approach they will adopt in solving the type of problem they are likely to encounter in the job.

Personality or psychometric testing

This measures individual characteristics which contribute to job performance. It is essential that expert training is obtained for those administering and feeding back test results. The maxim *caveat emptor* applies here because a number of ill-trained organizations offer packages of dubious validation.

The Institute of Personnel and Development can provide a fact sheet and more information about companies offering these services, if requested.

Candidates need to be informed in advance if job-related tests are to be used. It should be explained that the assessment is based on the person specification, and many organizations send this document to shortlisted candidates so that the criteria against which they are being selected is not blind. Constructive feedback should be given after the final selection has been made, in order for candidates to feel it was a positive experience from which they learned something to carry to the next interview, even if they have not got the job.

THE INTERVIEW   Many employers enter this process without much preparation and are surprised when the interview did not reveal all they thought it should or when, some months later, disconcerting things are discovered in the performance of the new appointee.

It is a fallacy to think that, because someone has the right qualifications and is able to show empathy with the views and experience of the interviewer, the person should be offered the job. This is an illustration of the mirror-image or halo effect to which we are all in danger of succumbing. We feel comfortable with people who are like us and tend to appoint such a person unless adequate groundwork has been done about skills and abilities needed for the particular job and the skills gap in the wider team. It should be appreciated that one might clash with one's closest friends if thrown together in a work situation.

It must also be realized that some people are natural sales-persons, regardless of their profession, and excel at selling themselves at interview, whilst others are more introverted and undersell themselves. The former category have a far better success record in an interview situation, but there is no correlation between selling oneself at interview and ability to do the job, unless, of course, the job is sales promotion! This demonstrates the inherent dangers of the interview process and can cloud the judgement of the interviewer(s) unless there is sufficient realization of these factors. Such factors can also be to the disadvantage of women and ethnic minorities, and undermine equal opportunities practices. Some ethnic minority candidates may not share common cultural backgrounds or experiences with the principals who might be interviewing them, and research demonstrates that women undersell themselves, compared with their male colleagues.

Awareness of all these factors will add to the objectivity of an inherently subjective process.

The guiding principle again, is to base the interview questions on the person specification and to appreciate exactly what elements of it can be tested in the interview situation, e.g. inter-personal skills, sensitivity, approach to problem solving, ability to react to on-the-spot difficult situations, long-term planning or strategy and persuasion. There are some simple but essential rules for conducting an interview.

Rules for conducting an interview

1. Where possible, have at least two interviewers. Two heads are better than one; the responsibility and assessment are shared and the process is (and is *seen* to be) more equitable. The more people who participate in decision making, the less potential for subsequent disagreement.
2. Ensure the right environment, i.e. the telephones are discon-nected/channelled elsewhere, the room is carefully laid out, e.g. do you want easy chairs or a desk in between you? Arrange

refreshment on arrival. Ensure that staff meeting candidates know their roles in the process.

3. Time-manage the interview and, if candidates wander off the point or dry up, bring them back to the focus of the question.

4. Have a standard set of points to explore, based on the person specification so that you can compare like with like, but first of all, set candidates at ease and achieve a rapport.

5. Maintain good eye contact. Do not glance at the clock, but place your watch somewhere you can glance at it discreetly.

6. Be an active listener, which means listening for approximately 80% of the time, and asking questions or explaining for approximately 20% of the time.

7. Make questions succinct and to the point. Do not combine two or three questions at once.

8. Do not become sidetracked by interesting red herrings. The fact that the candidate might rear chickens for free-range eggs should only be a useful 'ice-breaker' and not the subject of subsequent conversation!

9. Do not ask questions of a personal or sensitive nature without very good reasons. For example, if the concern is that someone is able to commence at reception promptly at 8.30 a.m., stress that this is an essential element of the job and ask if they are able to comply with this requirement. Do not ask if they have a young family and then make assumptions on the information given. Even if a candidate is turned down through sound reasons, to ask questions which are not job related leaves an employer open to potential challenges on the grounds of discrimination.

10. Take notes either during the interview or immediately after. You cannot objectively hope to remember the detailed responses after two candidates. This is the value of more than one interviewer. The person asking questions can maintain eye contact whilst another notes the responses in order to compare like with like afterwards.

11. Use a checklist which records responses to questions against the essentials of the person specification. This has already been agreed and makes the subsequent interpretation of answers and decision making a far more harmonious and consensual approach than might otherwise be the case.

IMPORTANCE OF AN INDUCTION PERIOD

Very often the employer fails to give adequate support to the new employee once he or she takes up the post, but the induction period is crucially important for both parties in defining and refining the 'misfits' of the selection procedure which quickly become apparent to both sides. It is not likely that the chosen candidate will be able to comply with all ideal aspects of the specification and be able to live up to the expectations of all in the practice. Similarly, after the initial honeymoon period is over, the chosen applicant will often have misgivings about what he or she has let himself or herself in for, and doubt their abilities to carry out all of the tasks to the extent of everyones expectations. The worst scenario is new staff being left to flounder in the mayhem of Monday morning in the practice!

There should, therefore, be an induction period of 6 months where a mentor (who may be a peer or a supervisor, but who plays the 'elder statesman' role) assists both the practice and the new recruit through this difficult process. During this period a need for further training in certain areas may emerge, and it is essential that any such needs are identified and addressed in the first 12 months, both for the smooth running of the practice and for the job satisfaction of the employee.

The selection process is important in this, because it should have highlighted any potential skill gaps to the employer, and through feedback, also to the employee. If development needs have not been identified through the selection process, subsequent short-comings can be damaging and demotivating for both parties.

The purpose of the selection methods is to identify any gaps between the best-fit candidate and the job, and to identify subsequently any training needs instead of to wait for these to manifest themselves as problems. Such a proactive approach yields positive results for both successful candidate and the practice.

MANAGING PERFORMANCE

Most doctors and other health care professionals would prefer to have nothing to do with correcting performance or attitude problems, but this is an integral part of the job for anyone who employs or supervises other people. Dealing with such 'people problems' can cause embarrassment and discomfort, and this in turn affects the skill with which the performance issue is handled, but skills can be developed in this area and simple procedures adopted which make the whole thing less subjective and uncomfortable.

It is useful to think of the word 'discipline' in its true meaning, i.e. education and learning, not in the punitive sense with which it is so often associated.

Effective action can contain problems and prevent them getting out of hand. The effectiveness of a partner or practice manager in this area can have a considerable impact on his or her relationships, not just with the person with the performance problems, but with the rest of the staff who will be demotivated if either the problems are not tackled or are tackled badly. In short, one performance problem not dealt with will mushroom into a number of other problems amongst team members.

Judgements have to be made about when to intervene and over what issues. Many people, including partners, have irritating habits that they cannot or will not change, and it may be pointless to try to make them. However, a balance must be struck because ignoring or being too lenient over issues may result in events getting out of hand; the analogy of a stitch in time saving nine can be highly appropriate with regard to discipline. Discrete action at the right time can prevent escalation into something far more difficult to contain. For this reason, things should never be allowed to drift. Prompt action should mean that dismissal is rarely necessary. This can be illustrated by a disciplinary pyramid (Figure 10.13). The base of the pyramid is the most important because, where there is effective first-line supervision, the ascending stages should never, or rarely be resorted to.

It is worth here defining the term 'counselling' to avoid confusion. It is not used in the context that would normally be understood by GPs, i.e. 'therapeutic counselling'. In the employment context, anyone who has a managing, supervising or mentoring role needs to develop counselling skills. It is an essential part of a manager's art to enable other people to develop their skills and effectiveness by helping them to find solutions to problems, thereby developing their own strengths and improving performance. It is particularly useful in dealing with performance problems and constitutes the first stage of the disciplinary procedure.

This section will look at the reasons for and nature of problems arising and how to conduct a proper appraisal review. It identifies the gap between required and actual performance, and will deal with how to confront performance problems and how to avoid common pitfalls. The law relating to this area of employment is also briefly explained and is dealt with in more detail in the chapter on

Figure 10.13
The disciplinary pyramid

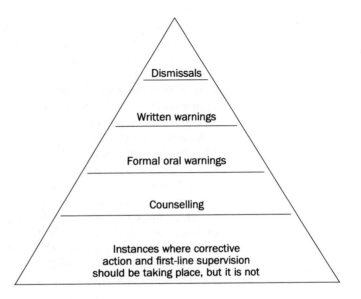

Source: Rees, W.D. (1996), *The Skills of Management.* International Thomson Press, London.

law. Many small employers, in particular, remain in blissful ignorance of the legal fundamentals until faced with a solicitor's letter on behalf of a former or even current employee.

Sample procedures and checklists are suggested, most of which are based on guidelines drawn up by ACAS, which offers a very useful free advice service on employment matters.

EFFECTIVE PERFORMANCE APPRAISAL   It is a well-researched and accepted fact that individuals are happiest and perform best when they can discuss frankly and be clear with their managers about:

◆ How they are performing.
◆ How their contribution is recognized.
◆ What they are expected to do in the future.
◆ How their employer will assist in their development.

Many GPs already communicate well with their staff and help them to maximize their performance on a day-by-day basis. However, even with the best will in the world, the best of communicators usually do not have the time to review staff performance effectively and constructively on an *ad hoc* basis. In this way, matters slip which should be addressed, the manager either does not notice or becomes used to less than satisfactory ways of working, and the employee regards less than satisfactory performance as the norm, perhaps without realizing the error of his or her ways.

A formal appraisal scheme is a cost-effective and time-effective way of ensuring staff motivation and performance, and of being able to deal with any problem areas at an embryonic stage.

This section looks at a framework for such an appraisal exercise.

Causes of failure   One of the most frequent causes of failure or dissatisfaction with a performance appraisal scheme is the fact that it seeks to fulfil many different and/or conflicting requirements. A clear impossibility is tying up salary considerations with a review of current performance. The problem is obvious: an appraisee will try to deny a failing or justify it if this failing is likely to have a direct effect on salary. Such a situation also places the manager in a very uncomfortable position. However, if the purpose of the discussion is to identify strengths as well as weak areas and look for ways in which these may be improved with no relation to pay, the appraisee is much more likely to participate openly and honestly in how performance might be improved.

Tying pay to performance has largely been discredited as a trend of business in the 1980s (Harvard Business Review, 1993) and has been demonstrated to damage team spirit, as well as the relationship between appraiser/appraisee. The single principle of improving current performance is now considered to be the most rewarding and justifiable purpose of a performance appraisal system.

When carried out properly, performance appraisal is an intensely valuable management tool in improving the individual and thus the practice. However, unless managers have the necessary skills to operate it, a performance appraisal system will become at best passive and of little value. At worst, it will be a minefield, disliked and feared by both parties alike. A bland interview aimed at avoiding real issues will add nothing to the employee's performance. A badly handled interview can cause conflict and alienation, and adversely affect the whole team. The manager conducting the interviews should, therefore, receive appropriate training.

As well as commercial organizations, health authorities will often provide such training for practice managers, and ACAS is an excellent source of 'best practice' and free advice.

The process suffers if the parties regard it as a 'once a year' exercise with no ongoing value throughout the year. A jointly agreed action plan and personal development plan should be reviewed regularly and updated in a less formal way than the annual interview, perhaps every 3 months.

These regular informal reviews provide an opportunity to check on progress, agree new or amended key objectives, and deal with problems as they arise.

CARRYING OUT PERFORMANCE APPRAISAL The action plan produced as a result of the appraisal expresses the agreement reached between the appraiser and appraisee in terms of 'key objectives' for the year ahead. Eight key objectives would be reasonable. Key objectives are not simply duties on the job description, but define key priorities for the next 12 months against which performance can be reviewed. Each key objective can be described as 'a statement of results to be achieved'. These could be:

♦ Task or service objectives.
♦ Management of resources (people, budgets, etc.).
♦ Personal effectiveness.

To be meaningful, objectives should be:

♦ Linked to the practice's objectives.
♦ Clear and specific.
♦ Important (i.e. worth monitoring).
♦ Challenging but achievable.
♦ Measurable in terms of results.
♦ Linked to a timescale.

In order to achieve this, the action plan requires both parties to record against each of the key objectives how they think the objectives can be achieved, the expected timescale and how they can judge when it has been achieved.

Tips for the appraiser or manager are:

♦ Invite the appraisee to 'lead off' the discussion based on the individual's preparation sheet which has been completed.
♦ Achievements must be recognized and acknowledged.
♦ The appraisee should be invited to explore her or his own weak areas before the manager's views are expressed.
♦ At all times the discussion must be positive and constructive with the emphasis on issues about which something can be done.
♦ Key objectives must be jointly agreed and recorded.
♦ A realistic development plan should be discussed and agreed.

Examples of the appraisal preparation sheet for both parties are shown in Figures 10.14 and 10.15.

Figure 10.14
Individual's preparation sheet

> The past year's work
>
> ♦ What do you feel were your main achievements and why?
> ♦ How well have you met the key objectives agreed at your last appraisal?
> ♦ What has caused you difficulty/what specific problems have you encountered in performing your job, and why?
>
> The coming year's work
>
> ♦ What do you want to achieve?
> ♦ How do you think you can meet these aims?
> ♦ How could you improve the way you work at present?
> ♦ How could you help yourself?
> ♦ How could your manager help you?
> ♦ What improvements could be made to the system in which you operate?

Figure 10.15
Manager's preparation sheet

> The past year's work
>
> ♦ What were her or his main achievements and why?
> ♦ How well has he or she met the key objectives agreed at your last appraisal?
> ♦ What has caused her or him difficulty/what specific problems has she or he encountered in performing the job and why?
>
> The coming year's work
>
> ♦ What do you want her or him to achieve?
> ♦ How do you think he or she can meet these aims?
> ♦ How could she or he improve the present ways of working?
> ♦ How could he or she help themselves?
> ♦ How could you help?
> ♦ Other issues needing discussion, e.g. improving work systems?

IDENTIFYING THE
PERFORMANCE
GAP

Careful selection, induction and appraisal should ensure the perfect performer, but sometimes performance problems will still arise...

The first thing is to establish that there really is a gap between required and actual performance. The gap is lessened the more we communicate with staff and there are many ways of communicating these duties and standards of performance that are expected. For example, through the contract of employment and job description, through 'on the job' and external training, through practice meetings or briefing sessions, through formal appraisal interviews, or on an informal individual basis. Procedures, standards and documentation such as job descriptions need to be up to date and communicated clearly.

Employees tend to be better motivated and more satisfied if they work within very clear guidelines, and this enhances creativity and initiative, not diminishes it. Protocols for expected performance in the day-to-day tasks of the practice should ideally be drawn up with the staff involved. This is part of effective practice development and can also be a very useful teambuilding exercise. Some of the best staff procedure manuals are produced in this way.

Information on actual performance can be gleaned from such sources as sickness and absence records, time-sheets, appraisal interviews, patient feedback or satisfaction surveys, and other staff within the practice. Comparison can also be made with others who perform similar tasks, e.g. is there any member of staff who attracts more complaints or who incurs more wastage, or who consistently fails to attain his or her own personal targets. Looking at what is expected and what has actually been achieved will establish whether a gap exists which needs closing.

In order to close the gap, we usually need to address one of, or a combination of, the four areas shown in Box 10.5.

Box 10.5
Reasons for problems
in performance

1. Personal issues that arise from domestic responsibilities and circumstances.
2. Practice management issues such as poor communication or procedures.
3. Personality or capability issues where the person is having difficulty in coping with the team or work requirements.
4. Where a complaint has been made about a member of the practice team.

Each of these areas are briefly explored below.

Personal issues

Domestic circumstances

These can include relationship problems, responsibility for child/elderly parent, being in a dual-career family, or financial or health problems.

Divorce or separation

This is one of the most frequent causes of stress which will impact directly on performance and work relationships. As it now occurs in more than one in three marriages, practices need to think through how to deal with this in a team situation.

Physical and mental ability

A health problem, perhaps as simple as eyesight, or stress connected with the above issues will affect an individual's ability to perform tasks.

Practice management issues

This covers a multitude of potential organizational pitfalls.

Poor management

Where the person's immediate supervisor is not adequately trained or does not offer the right degree of support. Lack of procedures or systems could be the problem, or inadequate communication between team members or inadequate information about what the job requires. Doctors' prime function is to spend their professional time being doctors, but this should not be to the exclusion of dedicating time to interpersonal relationships and building performance efficiency within the practice. This all contributes to patient care.

Inadequate job specification

People often do not appreciate exactly what is expected of them, or the job is simply too much for one person. New members of the team are often expected to 'slot in' without prior appreciation of the prevailing culture and ways of doing things in that particular practice. New blood can invigorate the practice as long as it is not expected to simply follow existing tradition and procedures which might not have been 'best practice' in the first place.

Change of job requirements

New technology, health authority requirements and the changing nature of primary care all place additional stress factors on the practice team. Where such changes are a difficult hurdle, this will result in lowered morale, motivation and performance. External factors and pressures are the most difficult to control and cope with, but they can be anticipated and planned, i.e. it enhances coping mechanisms and motivation to be proactive rather than reactive to such pressures.

Poor planning
Underperformance can result as a lack of direction and planning. Practice objectives and planning should be reflected in each individual's personal objectives as a result of the appraisal process. Planning needs to be realistic as opposed to idealistic and targets need to be achievable if they are not going to demotivate staff.

Poor induction and training
Before internal or external training takes place, induction plays a crucial role in the satisfactory assimilation of the new member of staff into the practice. Culture and style differs considerably between practices, as it does between any other organization. This needs to be absorbed by the newcomer at the same time as embarking on a training programme, the most important element of which will be internal on-the-job training to reinforce practice procedures and values.

Personality or capability issues A mismatch between the organization and the individual can be eliminated greatly by good selection and recruitment procedures. However, the following issues can still arise. A clash of personality or bad group dynamics – even the best recruitment practices will not always reveal an uncomfortable 'teamplayer' who does not share information readily and who communicates on a need-to-know basis. The nature and danger of group dynamics means that such a person may quickly become ostracized by the rest of the team, and this will aggravate the assimilation of that person and impede practice cohesion.

Conflict on moral or religious values
Ideological differences may result in some people being reluctant to work on the Sabbath of their particular religion or to participate in certain procedures such as assisting in termination of pregnancy. Such issues, where compliance to normal practice routines is required, should be made clear in the selection procedure so that a subsequent mismatch does not materialize, causing stress to the individual and to the rest of the team.

Inappropriate levels of confidence
An individual with too much confidence, above the level of experience, can be even more damaging than the unassertive underconfident person who initiates little of his or her own accord. Both situations require careful counselling, training and monitoring.

Intellectual ability
This may be inadequate for the job either because of a poor recruitment procedure, or because the nature of the job has changed and new demands are being made.

Complaints about a member of the practice team

A complaint from a patient or third party can, if handled badly, destroy self-confidence and relationships at work, therefore impairing performance. It is essential that a practice-based complaints procedure is in operation which complies with health authority requirements. Communication within the practice and with the complainant is a key in preventing an escalation of a complaint to formal stages. A laid-down and well-known procedure should ensure communication and strict time limits, but it is also essential that the staff member concerned receives proper mentoring and support from other team members. If an underlying cause or problem exists, such issues are best addressed quickly and locally, avoiding formal proceedings where possible.

Now that the reason for problems in performance have been explored, ways of tackling both the issues and the poor performer will be explained.

Figure 10.16
Ways of dealing with the poor performer

The following are not given in order of execution but as starting points to assist thinking when a problem arises:

♦ Good communication
  – Jointly agree specific, reasonable goals, and a date to review the performance.
♦ Training
  – Make sure you give appropriate training, preferably on the job, so there is no problem in making the connection between the training and the working situation.
♦ Dissatisfactions
  – Fill the gap where appropriate; remedy particular problems such as pay or conditions.
♦ Discipline
  – These range from the informal discussion through to increasingly formal procedures and punishment ultimately including dismissal.
♦ Reorganizing
  – Where the problem has arisen through difficulties with the work materials; reporting relationships; physical arrangements being no longer adequately organized.
♦ Management
  – Improve the clarity of communicating the task, monitoring systems or the expertise of a particular manager.
♦ Outside agencies
  – Particularly appropriate where there are personal and family reasons.
♦ The job
  – Transfer to a more appropriate job or department; redesign the job.
♦ Peer pressure
  – Where an individual performance is very different from the average, those working alongside will feel it inappropriate and may put pressure on the individual to change.

Source: Torrington *et al.* (1985), *Management Methods*, Institute of Personnel and Development, London.

Figure 10.17 gives examples of the kinds of problems which might arise and which need to be covered by rules.

Figure 10.17
The nature of problems
arising

◆ Time-keeping
  – What rules apply to lateness? In the absence of rules it can become at
    best a tolerated norm and, at worst, a serious demotivator for other
    members of staff.
◆ Absence
  – Who authorizes absence and approves holidays? To whom and when
    should employees notify their absence? In what circumstances will self-
    certification not be acceptable.
◆ Health and safety
  – What special requirements exist regarding personal appearance or
    cleanliness, e.g. length of hair, jewellery, protective clothing. Are there
    clear rules regarding special hazards or procedures, smoking and
    alcohol?
◆ Use of company facilities
  – Are private telephone calls permitted, or is any item of practice
    equipment permitted to leave the premises, or to be available for
    personal use?
◆ Discrimination
  – Is it clear that any form of racial or sexual abuse or harassment will be
    treated as disciplinary offences? Are there any rules about clothing
    which could be disadvantageous to a racial group?
◆ Gross misconduct
  – Are the kind of offences regarded as gross misconduct and which could
    lead to dismissal without notice, clearly specified? Example, theft or
    serious health and safety breaches.

HOW TO CONFRONT PERFORMANCE PROBLEMS

A problem that is confronted quickly will usually be well on the way to becoming solved. Here are some examples of situations where confronting is probably the only answer:

◆ When performance deteriorates and the person seems unhappy and unable to perform as usual.
◆ when the individual is disrupting the work group's performance in a way which affects the quality of other people's work.
◆ Persistently poor time-keeping.
◆ When counselling alone does not solve the problem. (N.B. Refer to page 260 for a definition of counselling in an employment context.)

A key to using the confronting of a problem positively is to recognize it as an opportunity to help an individual to develop professionally or personally. It is a way of enabling them to confront the problem, and offers them an opportunity to change and to find new ways of contributing to the success of the practice.

More often than not, immediate action at the counselling stage will prevent the problem developing further. This can be an opportunity for joint problem-solving and goal-setting, which is not the same as giving advice, but is much more effective because it enables the individual to 'own' the solution which is then more likely to be permanent. The best practitioners at this will enable other people to develop their abilities through finding their own solution to a problem. The most crucial skill needed for this is an ability to listen attentively without making premature assumptions and without being tempted to leap in with advice, or to glance at the clock on the wall. The room in which any such interview takes place needs to be free from interruption and any telephone needs to be disconnected.

There are different strategies for using this as a method for improving people's performance, but one successful formula is given in Figure 10.18.

Figure 10.18
Stages in a counselling interview

1. Factual interchange
   - Focus on the facts of the situation first. Ask factual questions and provide factual information, like the doctor asking about the location of the pain and other symptoms, rather than demonstrating dismay. This provides a basis for later analysis.
2. Opinion interchange
   - Open the matter up for discussion by asking for the employee's opinions and feelings, but not offering any criticism, nor making any decisions. Gradually, the matter is better understood by both parties.
3. Joint problem-solving
   - Ask the employee to analyse the situation described. Offer help in questioning and focus, but it must be the employee's own analysis, with the manager resisting the temptation to produce answers.
4. Decision-making
   - The manager helps to generate alternative lines of action for consideration and both parties share in deciding what to do. Only the employee can behave differently, but the manager may be able to help a change in behaviour by facilitation.

AVOIDING COMMON PITFALLS

Dealing with performance problems and particularly with the long-term poor performer can be one of the most difficult management situations to face. There are some common pitfalls which can be avoided, once they are known. These can include:

1. Not seeking help and handling a disciplinary matter on your own, particularly if you have little prior experience in this area. Guidance and advice can be obtained free from the Industrial Relations Officers at the Regional BMA offices (available only to members), or from the regional ACAS offices. Some health authorities may also be prepared to offer management advice.
2. Not checking out existing practice procedures, or not having adequate procedures to follow in the first place. Use procedures based on ACAS guidance and follow them meticulously.
3. Not keeping a record. Records of any conversation or interview connected with performance, need to be kept for two reasons. Firstly, it is impossible to subsequently recall things accurately. Secondly, if the problems persist, the claims that an individual has been counselled and subsequently warned can be denied.

Box 10.6
Checklist for dealing with poor performance

The following checklist is designed to help you to consider the factors involved in confronting problems constructively and to help assess your performance when you do. Consider each answer carefully.

	Yes, I do this well	I do this, but I would like to improve my performance	No, I need to improve my performance as a matter of priority
Do you pay close attention to staff who have recently taken on new duties?	☐	☐	☐
Do you give staff clear and regular feedback on their performance?	☐	☐	☐
Do you confront the individual in question rather than complain to colleagues?	☐	☐	☐
Do you express yourself clearly and concisely to the individual you are confronting?	☐	☐	☐
Do you stress the importance of finding a solution to the problem?	☐	☐	☐
Do you suggest positive ways of resolving the problem?	☐	☐	☐
Are you prepared to understand, although not necessarily agree with, the person's point of view?	☐	☐	☐
Do you deal with the situation calmly but sensitively?	☐	☐	☐
Do you avoid the trap of using the situation as an excuse to unload your own frustration on someone else?	☐	☐	☐

4. Acting too hastily. Whilst all performance problems need to be nipped in the bud promptly, never make snap decisions. The implications of any action need to be carefully thought out. In the most extreme cases, if it is felt necessary that a member of staff should not be on the premises, that person can be suspended and sent home which allows any emotional or high

feelings to subside and allows the proper procedures to be checked out.

5. Acting inconsistently. This will be noticed by other members of staff, who will feel demotivated as a result. It is also potentially unlawful to apply different standards, expectations or punishments to different staff. This is why having proper, simple procedures are so important. Not only are they objective and fair, but they are seen to be fair.

6. Not listening thoroughly to the 'other side' or having made your mind up about a problem situation in advance. This will severely jeopardize the chances of a successful outcome and showing this attitude of mind is likely to increase any antagonism in the other party.

7. Concentrating on personality issues instead of the facts. One of the most useful rules of negotiating is to be hard on the issues but soft on the person. This will help to prevent an emotionally charged situation developing and will help you to feel firmly in control.

8. Trying to avoid dealing with the issue. Tackling a performance problem in a colleague is never easy, but a problem not dealt with rarely disappears and usually becomes far worse and proportionately more difficult to handle, as was illustrated in the 'disciplinary pyramid' (Figure 10.13).

The questions shown in Box 10.6 (p. 262) illustrate some important considerations in how to approach dealing with poor performance. The checklist could be a useful aid in planning how to tackle a problem and where there is room for improvement.

PERFORMANCE PROBLEMS AND THE LAW

The need for contracts and a disciplinary policy

UK law requires that employers provide employees with a written grievance and disciplinary policy attached to the contract of employment within 8 weeks of starting work. Although this only applies to those working at least 8 hours a week, exclusions should not be relied upon for two reasons:

1. As already demonstrated, there are clear benefits to supplying all employees with guidelines about the job requirements and standards of performance expected of them.

2. The chapter on statutory and legal responsibilities has made clear that employment law is a rapidly evolving area. It is, therefore, to the advantage and protection of the employer to provide common rights and policies for all, wherever possible.

Unfair dismissal and employer's defences

Regardless of the number of hours worked, an employee with 2 years service is entitled to make a claim to an industrial tribunal for unfair dismissal within 3 months of the end of their employment.

However, this is something no practice need fear if it has followed the guidance in this chapter and adheres to the ACAS

Figure 10.19
Disciplinary procedure

1. Purpose and scope
The Company's aim is to encourage improvement in individual conduct. This procedure sets out the action which will be taken when disciplinary rules are breached.

2. Principles
(a) The procedure is designed to establish the facts quickly and to deal consistently with disciplinary issues. No disciplinary action will be taken until the matter has been fully investigated.
(b) At every stage employees will have the opportunity to state their case and be represented, if they wish, at the hearings by a shop steward, if appropriate, or by a fellow employee.
(c) An employee has the right to appeal against any disciplinary penalty.

3. The procedure
◆ *Stage 1 – Oral warning:* If conduct or performance is unsatisfactory, the employee will be given a formal oral warning, which will be recorded. The warning will be disregarded after ... months satisfactory service.
◆ *Stage 2 – Written warning:* If the offence is serious, if there is no improvement in standards, or if a further offence occurs, a written warning will be given which will include the reason for the warning and a note that, if there is no improvement after ... months, a final written warning will be given.
◆ *Stage 3 – Final written warning:* If conduct or performance is still unsatisfactory, a final written warning will be given, making it clear that any recurrence of the offence or other serious misconduct within a period of ... months will result in dismissal.
◆ *Stage 4 – Dismissal:* If there is no satisfactory improvement or if further serious misconduct occurs, the employee will be dismissed.

4. Gross misconduct
If, after investigation, it is confirmed that an employee has committed an offence of the following nature (the list is not exhaustive), the normal consequence will be dismissal:

◆ Theft.
◆ Damage to company property.
◆ Fraud.
◆ Incapacity for work due to being under the influence of alcohol or illegal drugs.
◆ Physical assault.
◆ Gross insubordination.

  While the alleged gross misconduct is being investigated, the employee may be suspended, during which time he or she will be paid the normal hourly rate. Any decision to dismissal will be taken by the employer only after a full investigation.

5. Appeals
An employee who wishes to appeal against any disciplinary decision must do so to the employer within 2 working days. The employer will hear the appeal and decide the case as impartially as possible.

Source: ACAS (1990)

guidelines which follow. Employers need to be aware that there is no time-qualifying period for claims on the grounds of discrimination against race, sex or disability, but, again, the same fair procedures applied to all staff, provide protection to employers.

Dismissals are generally not unfair if on the grounds of misconduct, capability, lack of qualification or redundancy. Incapability can be justified because of a person's poor performance or on medical grounds. Misconduct can be justified on the grounds of either a single act of gross misconduct, which entitles an employer to dismiss without notice, or because of cumulative misconduct, where the appropriate notice period or money in lieu must be given.

Dismissal due to absence record   Employment can be terminated because of a bad sickness absence record on the grounds of:

1. Capability – where there is an underlying chronic condition;
2. Conduct – where there is no underlying chronic condition, in which case dismissal is on the grounds of an unacceptable absence level (regardless of whether the unconnected illness are genuine or not).

Whilst the practice will obviously want to afford as much support as possible to a member of staff suffering from ill-health, there might come a time when the level of absence is unacceptable to the normal running of the practice and service to patients, or is placing an undue strain on other members of staff. In this situation, one of the above procedures need to be followed in a sensitive and supportive manner.

Figure 10.19 shows a sample ACAS guideline for a disciplinary procedure in a small firm. It can be adjusted to suit individual practices, but the principles apply to any business and provide protection against legal action if the procedures are carried out fairly.

It should be noted that it must be apparent in the procedures who is responsible for taking disciplinary action, not least because such staff need a clear understanding of, and preferably training, in this area of management. The Practice Manager would normally fulfil this role for support staff, with the right of appeal being to one of the Partners. Ideally a Partner should wear a 'staffing hat' in order to develop experience and some expertise in an area where consistency is absolutely vital.

CONCLUSION   At least 70% of total management costs in general practice is the 'people management' factor. Considerable and largely unrealized savings can be made in this area by simply applying tried and tested procedures and processes, thereby accumulating the necessary experience and skills. The best of procedures 'stand alone' and are ineffective without the interpersonal skills needed to operate them.

The shift from secondary to primary care can be viewed either as an opportunity or a threat by general practitioners and the primary

care team. The proactive approach (as opposed to simply responding to political dictats) is to seize the opportunity and recruit and
develop staff to take the practice in a planned direction.

In general practice, there is still a prevailing trend to appoint on
the basis of an interview only. This has been demonstrated to be
unsound, with a disproportionate cost/risk factor. Alternative
techniques have been explored and explained which are relatively
simple and cost effective.

The procedures described may at first perusal seem time
consuming but, when practised regularly, will become 'business as
usual', and in the long run will save not only time, but also money,
because the cost of a single mistake in the recruitment process is
enormous to the practice.

Human resource planning is a poor relation, if carried out at all,
to business planning. Yet the success of the business plan rests on
the ability of the human resources plan to implement it. It is
amazing that often more effort goes into a major capital investment,
such as a new information technology system, than into the people
needed to operate, implement and interpret it. In this respect, a leaf
could be taken out of the Japanese book of management, where
corporate planning starts with the people and a skills audit.

Performance management is an area which attracts more attention and rhetoric than applied practice and attention to detail. This
area particularly requires sound procedures, tools and skills to
operate effectively. It is equally easy to get it right as wrong, but to
get it wrong can result in lowered morale, bad performance and, at
worst, legal sanctions. The chapter has explored, in some depth,
how to get it right.

As general practice expands into a primary care-led business, it is
essential that these factors are realized and translated into the
business planning process. To do so will result in a better work
environment and a competitive advantage.

SUMMARY

People management in general practice needs to be thought of in
terms of a 'cradle to grave' approach, starting with the business
plan and then deciding on the competencies of people needed to
implement if successfully. This involves human resource planning,
which identifies the gap between what is in place and what is
needed.

Filling the gap involves translating these competencies into
something that can be identified and measured for both incoming
and existing staff. This is normally easier to do with staff joining the
practice (as long as stringent recruitment procedures are followed)
than for existing employees.

Recruitment procedures should be objective and ensure a 'best
fit', followed up by an induction period in which training needs are
identified and addressed.

Performance needs to be monitored through an appropriate appraisal system which is 'user friendly' to both parties. Performance problems thereafter need to be dealt with in accordance with recognized protocols and need to be seen to be both explicit and reasonable. ACAS guidelines should be consulted before termination of a contract.

Interpersonal skills are the crucial success element in the above procedures, and need to be acquired by all those with a supervisory or management role to play.

FURTHER READING

♦ ACAS (1991), *Employing People: A Handbook for Small Firms*. Advisory handbook. ACAS, London.

♦ ACAS (1992), *Discipline at Work*. Advisory handbook. ACAS, London.

♦ ACAS (1993), *Recruitment and Induction*. Advisory booklet. ACAS, London.

♦ ACAS (1993), *Employment Policies*. Advisory booklet. ACAS, London.

These ACAS publications are part of a series of handbooks and advisory booklets which give the best possible advice on all aspects of employment. They are essentially practical, providing checklists, codes of practice and specimen procedures and letters At only £2 each, they are 'a must' for every employers bookcase!

♦ Belbin, M. (1994), *Team Roles At Work*. Butterworth/Heinemann, Oxford.

♦ Rees, W.D. (1996), *The Skills of Management*. International Thomson Press, London.

This book is an excellent theory-based but practical introduction to management, dealing with the case skills essential to modern management. David Rees has the gift of being able to summarize considerable learning in an accessible and even entertaining way.

♦ Weightman, J. (1993), *Managing Human Resources*. The Institute of Personnel and Development, London.

This book explains communication and learning, and shows how they can be applied in practice. It deals with a broad range of personnel issues, particularly motivation and performance management.

REFERENCES

ACAS (1995), *Recruitment Policies for the 1990s*, Advisory booklet. ACAS, London.

ACAS (1990), *Discipline at Work*, Advisory handbook. ACAS, London.

Conference calls for changes in medical education. *British Medical Journal* **307**: 168.

Kohn, A. (1993), Why incentive plans cannot work. *Harvard Business Review* Sept–October.

Rees, W.D. (1996), *The Skills of Management*. International Thomson Press, London.

Snowise, N.G. (1992), General practice partnerships: till death us do part? *British Medical Journal, General Practice* **305**: 398–400.

Torrington, D., Weightman, J. and Johns, K. (1985), *Management Methods*, Institute of Personnel Management, London.

Weightman, J. (1993), *Managing Human Resources*. The Institute of Personnel and Development, London.

USEFUL CONTACTS   ACAS (Advisory, Conciliation and Arbitration Service)
Brandon House
180 Borough High Street
London, UK

Equal Opportunities Commission
Overseas House
Quay Street
Manchester, UK

Commission for Racial Equality
Elliot House
10–12 Allington Street
London, UK

Institute of Personnel and Development
IPD House
Camp Road
London, UK

British Medical Association
BMA House
Tavistock Square
London, UK

INDEX

Note: text in Boxes, Figures and Tables is indicated by *italic page numbers*. Index entries are arranged in letter-by-letter order (ignoring spaces).